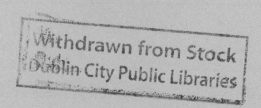

Deliciously Healthy
Menopause

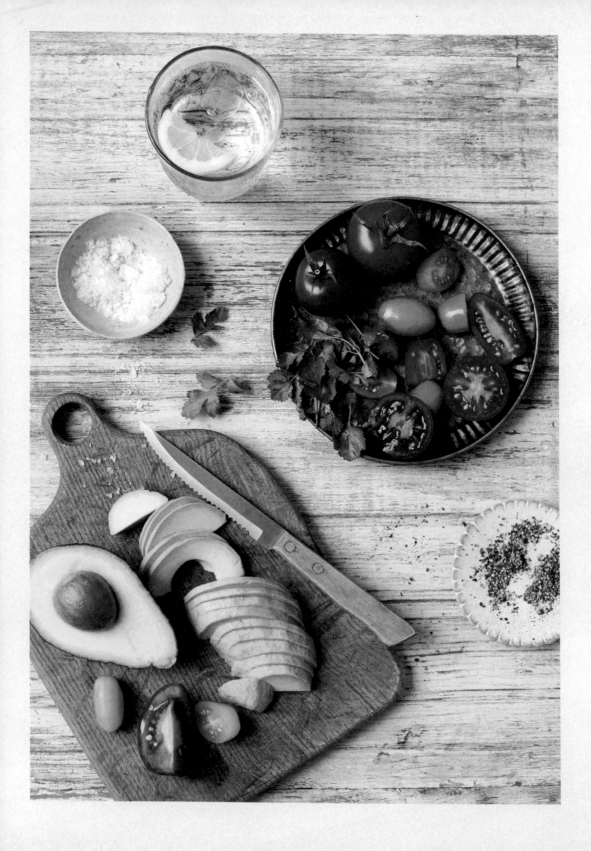

Deliciously Healthy
Menopause

Food and recipes for optimal health throughout
the perimenopause and menopause

Leabharlanna Chathair Bhaile Átha Cliath
Dublin City Libraries

SEVERINE MENEM

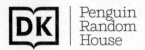

Project Editor	Claire Cross
Project Designers	Emma Forge and Tom Forge
Senior Editor	Dawn Titmus
Senior Designer	Barbara Zuniga
Editor	Kiron Gill
Editorial Assistant	Charlotte Beauchamp
Jacket Designer	Amy Cox
Jacket Coordinator	Lucy Philpott
Senior Production Editor	Tony Phipps
Senior Producer	Luca Bazzoli
Creative Technical Support	Sonia Charbonnier
Managing Editor	Dawn Henderson
Managing Art Editor	Marianne Markham
Art Director	Maxine Pedliham
Publishing Director	Katie Cowan
Photographer	Luke Albert
Food and Prop Stylist	Libby Silbermann

Disclaimer, see page 224

First published in Great Britain in 2022 by
Dorling Kindersley Limited
DK, One Embassy Gardens, 8 Viaduct Gardens,
London, SW11 7BW

The authorised representative in the EEA is
Dorling Kindersley Verlag GmbH.
Arnulfstr. 124, 80636 Munich, Germany

A CIP catalogue record for this book
is available from the British Library.
ISBN: 978-0-2415-3718-3

Printed and bound in China

For the curious
www.dk.com

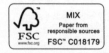

Contents

Preface

We live in a wonderful time when the menopause is no longer taboo in many parts of the world. The reality of the menopause is often shared in the media, from articles in mainstream news outlets, to the BBC campaign, *Wake Up to the Menopause*. Excellent charities, such as Daisy Network and The Menopause Charity, inform women on what is happening in the menopause and what they can do about it. Corporates are launching menopause initiatives to support their employees, and secondary school students are being taught about the menopause. Women in midlife no longer have to go through the menopause alone.

Despite this flow of information, the message often remains the same: the menopause is a miserable transition in a woman's life with terrible symptoms, for which the only solution is HRT. Although beneficial, HRT is not a magic pill and is not always easily accessible to every woman: from getting an appointment quickly, to contraindications to taking HRT, to actually being prescribed HRT and being able to receive it (there have been chronic shortages of some types), women can encounter obstacles. Furthermore, HRT doesn't always resolve all menopausal symptoms.

   More surprisingly, most women readily acknowledge they would rather try something natural before taking HRT. They often find, though, that there is too little information on natural approaches or that information is hard to access, so they turn to HRT.

There are a number of natural solutions that can help with symptoms. As a nutritional therapist specializing in the menopause, I can help midlife women improve their health, so they in turn lose weight and find relief from their symptoms. Nutritional therapy focuses on the principle that health can be achieved through a holistic and personalized approach to nutrition and lifestyle. Health comes from looking after our nutrition, sleep, fitness, and stress levels.

It is not emphasized enough that women can have an easy menopause; in fact, studies suggest that about one in four women do. The earlier you prepare, the more likely you are to have an easy, or easier, transition. The menopause tends to make existing conditions worse, so addressing concerns ahead of the menopause and/or updating your lifestyle is very likely to result in positive outcomes. It's never too late to start making positive changes.

While each woman is different, I'm aiming to make this book accessible to everyone who wants to understand why and how they can amend their diet and lifestyle to best prepare for or help with the menopause. The delicious recipes in the book are ones that the whole family can enjoy and include ingredients to help alleviate symptoms and optimize health. It's an holistic approach and consistency will yield the best results, giving you an excellent foundation for a healthy menopause.

Food is life, so I hope you enjoy my colourful and flavoursome recipes, inspired by my travels around the world. The menopause can be very enjoyable, we just need to make it work for ourselves.

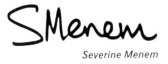

Severine Menem

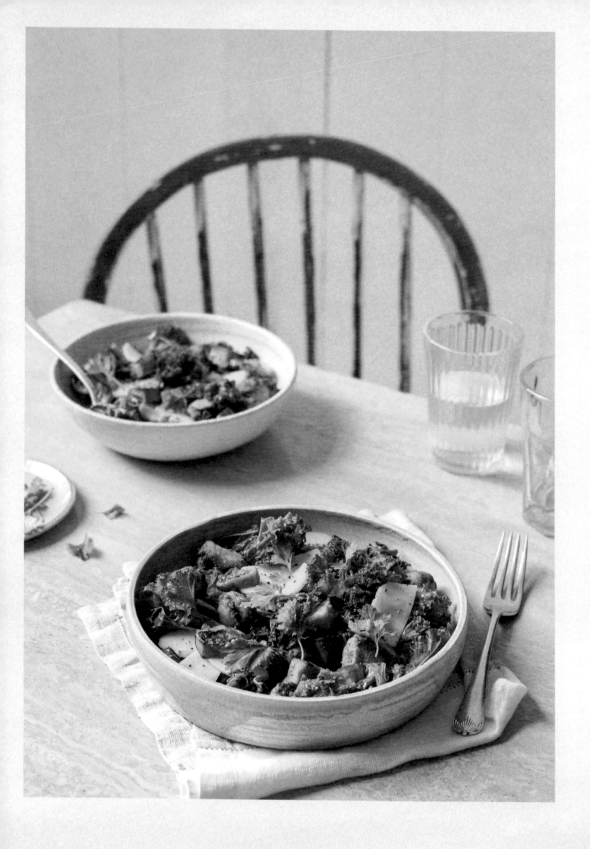

Living well
for the menopause

The menopause years

The menopause is a natural transition in a woman's life. Officially, the menopause is defined as not having had a period for 12 months, but reaching this point is a gradual process that can take place over a number of years. Understanding what is happening to your hormones and body during this time, the symptoms you may experience, and what you can do about them can help you put in place lifestyle measures to cope and enjoy a good quality of life in the menopause and beyond.

Why does the menopause happen?

The menopause is triggered by a low number of eggs in the ovaries, which impacts the production of oestrogen and other sex hormones. The fluctuations in these hormones and their varying ratios cause most menopausal symptoms (see pp.14–17). In the UK, the average age for the menopause is 51, although it is common for women to go through the menopause anywhere between the ages of 45 and 55.

The perimenopause

This describes the period leading up to the menopause, which can last for several years. During this time, egg stores drop and ovarian hormone levels fluctuate randomly, initiating changes in the menstrual cycle and, often, the onset of menopausal symptoms. Menstrual changes vary considerably between women, with periods becoming longer or shorter, heavier or lighter, and more or less frequent. For most women, the perimenopause heralds the onset of menopausal symptoms, typically vasomotor symptoms such as hot flushes and night sweats, which 80 per cent of women experience. Usually these occur for four years after the last menstrual period but they can last much longer. Although the chances are very low, it is still possible to become pregnant now so contraception should continue to be used.

The menopause and post-menopause

The point 12 months after the last menstrual period (without using contraception) marks the official end of a woman's natural reproductive life, when she is menopausal and enters post-menopause. While menopausal symptoms typically last for about four years after the end of menstruation for most women, they can continue for up to 12 years for around 10 per cent of women.

Premature and early menopause

Around 5 per cent of women experience the menopause between the ages of 40 and 45, known as early menopause.

For a very small number of women, the menopause takes place before their forties – in their thirties or, rarely, in their twenties or earlier. This is referred to either as premature menopause, premature ovarian failure, or primary ovarian insufficiency (POI). Around 1 per cent of women experience a spontaneous POI, often with no known cause, which can be extremely hard to cope with psychologically. Some known causes of POIs include autoimmune diseases and inherited conditions, such as galactosaemia. An increasing number of women enter premature menopause as a result of surgery (the removal of one or two ovaries and/or the uterus) and cancer treatments such as chemotherapy or radiotherapy, which can have a damaging effect on the ovaries.

Your hormones now

Hormones are messengers that play an important role in the body, regulating many essential functions. Changes to hormone levels in midlife cause many of the symptoms of the menopause and, together with the effects of ageing, can impact long-term health.

Oestrogen

There are three types of this female sex hormone: oestrone, oestradiol, and oestriol. Oestradiol is the most potent and prevalent in women from puberty up until the menopause; oestrone is the primary form of oestrogen after the menopause, and oestriol is produced during pregnancy by the placenta. Oestrogen helps to control the menstrual cycle, supports bone health, improves muscle mass and strength, protects heart health, supports brain function, and helps regulate mood.

- **What happens at the menopause?** Oestrogen starts to fall and randomly fluctuate after the age of 35, before levels plummet at the menopause. Its decline leads to symptoms such as hot flushes, night sweats, mood swings, and vaginal dryness. Lower levels increase the risk of cardiovascular disease and also affect how the body responds to insulin, making it harder to control blood sugar levels so increasing the possibility of diabetes. Lower oestrogen also affects bone density, raising the risk of osteoporosis post-menopause.

Progesterone

This female sex hormone helps to regulate the menstrual cycle and to maintain pregnancy.

- **What happens at the menopause?** Progesterone levels start to drop in our mid-thirties, before oestrogen starts to fall, and continue to decline in perimenopause. Low progesterone leads to irregular or absent periods.

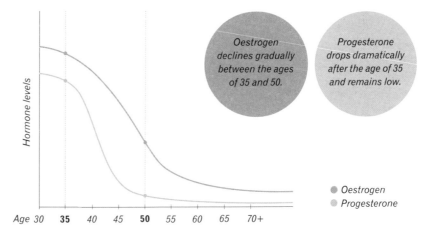

Female sex hormones

At the menopause, oestrogen drops but remains fairly steady and relatively high in comparison to progesterone.

Oestrogen declines gradually between the ages of 35 and 50.

Progesterone drops dramatically after the age of 35 and remains low.

Hormone levels

Age 30   **35**   40   45   **50**   55   60   65   70+

● Oestrogen
● Progesterone

Testosterone

This sex hormone plays an important role in libido and sexual health, promotes strong bones, and helps us to feel energized.

• **What happens at the menopause?** Although its decline is relatively small, lower levels can affect libido, mood, and energy levels.

Other hormones

Cortisol, the stress hormone, is produced by the adrenal glands. The right amount helps to regulate blood sugar and blood pressure. In the menopause, the adrenal glands start to become responsible for the production of some hormones, such as oestrogen and progesterone. If not looked after and/or under chronic stress, they overproduce cortisol.

Insulin helps to keep our blood sugar levels within a healthy range. As we age, we are more likely to become insulin resistant because of hormonal fluctuations and because insulin receptors work less efficiently. A high sugar diet exacerbates these problems. Our bodies continue to produce insulin, which remains in the blood, leading to diabetes and weight gain.

The thyroid gland produces endocrine hormones that are responsible for a healthy metabolism. Some symptoms of thyroid disease, such as weight gain and low energy, may be incorrectly attributed to the menopause. Lower oestrogen levels can also impact the thyroid, so it is important to test thyroid function if you are concerned.

Menopausal symptoms

While some women suffer few menopausal symptoms, this transition can bring a range of symptoms for many, impacting women's personal and professional lives.

How women are affected

There are at least 40 menopause symptoms. These can be physical, mental, and psychological. They can also affect all the body's systems.

Changes to the menstrual cycle, affecting frequency, duration, and/or flow, are often the first symptoms of the menopause. These can happen with or without other symptoms. On average, women experience seven symptoms, the most common two being hot flushes and vaginal dryness. Hot flushes are frequently discussed, but vaginal dryness is just as common and so it is important not to neglect this symptom. While there are many ways to deal with hot flushes, which eventually disappear, vaginal dryness has fewer remedies and can often become permanent if not treated.

Menopausal symptoms can last from just a few months to several years. On average, women experience symptoms over a period of 4–8 years, starting in the perimenopause, though for some they may go on for longer (see p.11). With a natural menopause, around 20 per cent of women have mild or no symptoms. Around 80 per cent of women experience symptoms, with 25 per cent of those suffering severe symptoms. Strong symptoms can be linked to genetics, general health, and menstrual history. Symptoms may also be stronger in women who have a natural menopause before the age of 45 or a menopause brought on by surgery or cancer treatment (see p.11).

It is important to address symptoms as soon as they appear, so that you can continue to enjoy your life personally and professionally.

Vasomotor symptoms

These symptoms are caused by the dilation or constriction of blood vessels. Our core body temperature usually remains within a set range, going up and down according to our circadian rhythm – the body's internal clock that governs its natural rhythms – the point we are at in our menstrual cycle, and any immune response. Hormonal fluctuations in the menopause can affect the temperature-controlling centre in the brain, leading to an exaggerated response by blood vessels.

- **Hot flushes** *are the most common vasomotor symptom. They start when blood vessels near the skin's surface widen to cool off, causing a sweat. Women feel a sensation of sudden heat, sometimes accompanied by redness, which may spread to the face and neck. There may be sweating and clammy skin.*
   Night sweats are hot flushes that occur while asleep, waking you up feeling hot and sweaty and making it hard to settle back to sleep. Both hot flushes and night sweats vary in frequency and intensity.

- **Cold flushes** *can occur when a hot flush fades, causing chills and shivering.*

- **Heart palpitations** *are felt by some women, either on their own or with hot flushes. These are experienced as a fluttering, pounding, or rapid heart rate.*

Urino-genitary symptoms

Falling oestrogen levels affect the lining of the uterus, vagina, and the bladder, causing tissues to thin and become less elastic and more sensitive. Localized issues such as vaginal dryness can affect libido.

- **Vaginal dryness** *is one of the most common menopause symptom. It tends to increase with age, with over 50–60 per cent of post-menopausal women affected. This is due exclusively to the drop in oestrogen at the menopause.*

- **Bladder issues** *include incontinence, as the pelvic floor weakens, and more frequent urinary tract infections (UTIs).*

Nervous and psychological symptoms

A combination of fluctuating hormone levels in the menopause, and how women respond to the various symptoms these can cause, can lead to the range of nervous and psychological symptoms shown here. Low libido can also be affected by physical symptoms such as vaginal dryness.

Insomnia *is common in the menopause. Heightened anxiety can mean women find it hard to fall asleep and wake frequently. An increased need to empty the bladder at night and night sweats exacerbate sleep problems. If broken nights are frequent and persistent, this adds to fatigue and impacts mood.*

Anxiety *may arise or worsen in the perimenopause. Women often wake in the night or early in the morning feeling anxious and may also have palpitations.*

Brain fog *describes the lack of focus, poor concentration, and faulty memory often experienced by women in the menopause.*

Irritability and mood swings *are common symptoms. Low energy levels, anxiety, and insomnia can all affect mood. The risk of depression rises now.*

Low libido *can result from a drop in oestrogen and progesterone. Other symptoms such as fatigue and low mood can contribute.*

Headaches *are commonly linked to fluctuating hormone levels. Stress, anxiety, and fatigue can also lead to menopausal headaches.*

Musculo-skeletal symptoms

Oestrogen is key for muscle and bones, so its decline during menopause impacts musculo-skeletal health. A poor lifestyle can mean that symptoms are felt more keenly. Hydration is also key – we absorb less water as we age, which is needed to lubricate the small fluid-filled sacs called bursae that prevent friction in joints.

Muscles *can feel tender, sore, and tense and aching muscles can impact sleep.*

Achy joints and muscles *are common in the menopause. Joints may feel stiffer on waking. Weight gain in the menopause can put additional pressure on the joints.*

A natural decline in bone density *with age is exacerbated by the drop in oestrogen, which can lead to osteoporosis postmenopause.*

Skin, hair, and nails

The drop in oestrogen impacts skin. It leads to a decline in collagen, which can mean that skin becomes drier and less elastic during the menopause. These changes can also make the skin more sensitive to products such as soaps and detergents, which can irritate the skin and cause itchiness. Hair and nails are also affected by a reduction in oestrogen.

Itchy skin *is common in the menopause, caused by low oestrogen levels that can lead to dry skin. Small bumps can appear on the surface of the skin and rashes may occur on the neck, chest, limbs, and back. Some women report a crawling sensation on the skin and tingling, prickling, or pins and needles-like numbness. Women may also experience menopausal acne.*

Changes to hair and nails *often occur now. Typically, hair thins and loses volume, though facial hair can increase. Fingernails may weaken and break easily.*

Digestion and weight gain

Hormonal changes impact digestion. The decline in oestrogen also leads to increased weight gain in the menopause.

Bloating, *indigestion, gas, constipation, and diarrhoea are more common. Existing problems such as IBS can worsen.*

Weight gain *is common, especially around the waist. An accumulation of fat here increases the risk of diabetes and cardiovascular disease in midlife.*

Other symptoms

Hormonal changes, particularly the fall in oestrogen, can also contribute to a range of other symptoms that become more common with age.

Sore breasts

Dry eyes

Changes to body odour and bad breath

Bleeding gums

Burning tongue or roof of mouth

Tinnitus and dizziness

Optimizing nutrition
for the menopause

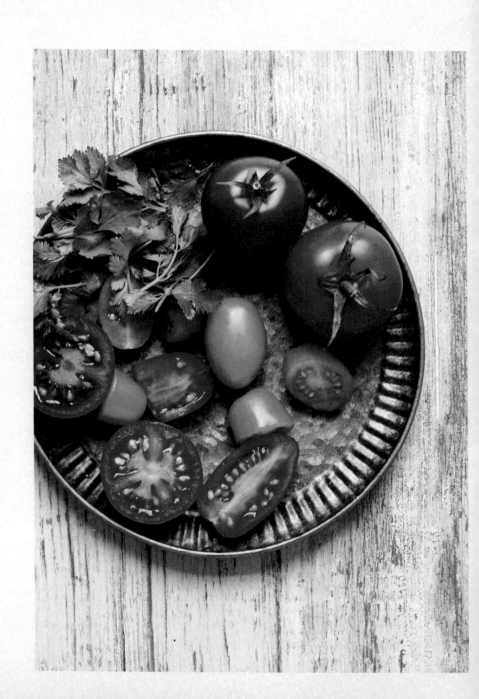

Good nutrition is the ideal throughout each stage of your life. When you eat well – ensuring your diet includes a healthy balance of the main food groups with a wide range of essential nutrients, and that you are adequately hydrated – your body and mind are energized and able to carry out vital functions, and your quality of life is enhanced.

As we approach midlife, and for women the menopause, what we eat becomes more important than ever. The combined effects of hormonal changes and natural ageing processes mean that your body has to work harder now and, subsequently, greater demands are placed on your nutrient stores. The following chapter sets out clearly your nutritional needs in this important period of transition, explaining exactly how getting the right amounts of each food group is paramount, which foods you should avoid, and how the healthy foods we eat and the host of micronutrients they provide have myriad benefits for body and mind throughout the menopause years.

Reviewing your diet for the menopause

The body is a wonderful machine – even if neglected for a number of years, it will often carry out its functions without much noticeable impact. However, as we approach midlife, visible changes such as easier weight gain indicate that the body is transitioning, and signpost a need to take stock of our diets and lifestyle if these have been less than optimal.

Adapting your diet now

As you approach the menopause, weight may be acquired more easily, skin may be less plump, sleep may be erratic, and you may develop anxiety. You may tire quickly, have less energy, and experience brain fog. All of these changes signal that your body is adapting. As a result, you may need to adjust your diet and lifestyle to meet your changing needs. Taking a positive approach to nutrition now can improve symptoms and help you manage concerns such as weight gain, which will positively impact your health long-term.

Getting sufficient nutrients

The way in which your body regulates itself as well as changes to hormone levels increase health risks in midlife. Optimizing nutrition now helps to lower the risk of osteoporosis, sarcopenia (muscle atrophy), neurological issues, and heart disease.

As you age, your body is less efficient at absorbing nutrients. In addition, heavy menstruation in the perimenopause can reduce minerals such as iron. These factors mean that women often enter the menopause with suboptimal nutrient levels, exacerbating symptoms and increasing

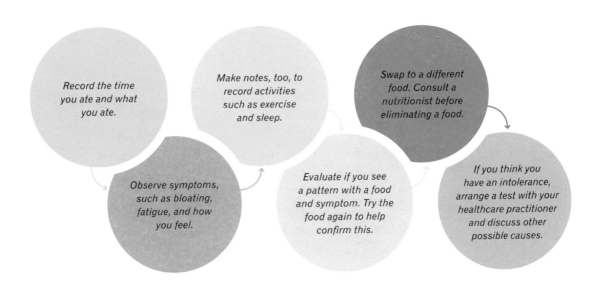

Record the time you ate and what you ate.

Observe symptoms, such as bloating, fatigue, and how you feel.

Make notes, too, to record activities such as exercise and sleep.

Evaluate if you see a pattern with a food and symptom. Try the food again to help confirm this.

Swap to a different food. Consult a nutritionist before eliminating a food.

If you think you have an intolerance, arrange a test with your healthcare practitioner and discuss other possible causes.

Keeping a food journal

This is the best way to be aware of what's happening in your body and to spot links between foods and how they worsen or help menopausal symptoms.

health risks. Other factors also impact nutrients. These include a decrease in stomach acid, which hampers calcium absorption; the skin's reduced ability to make vitamin D; and certain diets and/or poor gut health, which can leave the body low in vitamin B12. A varied, healthy diet, as outlined on pages 22–47, helps to optimize health in midlife.

Thinking about bioavailability

Although a food may be high in a nutrient, this does not mean that the body absorbs the nutrient easily, known as bioavailability. For example, nonheme iron (in plant foods) is less readily absorbed than heme iron (in animal foods). Nonheme iron can be blocked by certain compounds, such as substances called phytates, found in grains, nuts, seeds, and legumes. Eating vitamin C with plant proteins helps iron absorption, and vegetarians need a varied diet to ensure a wide intake of nutrients. Other ways to help the absorption of nutrients include cooking tomatoes to release lycopene and using oil and fats to absorb fat-soluble vitamins A, D, E, and K. The varied recipes in this book help you maximize your absorption of nutrients.

Staying nourished in the menopause

Each of us has individual nutritional needs as our bodies are affected by factors such as our genes, which can impact nutrient absorption; our environment, which may increase our need for antioxidants; whether we have developed food allergies or intolerances, which are more common with age; and our lifestyle and general health. While a qualified nutritionist can help to personalize your diet, there are some general guidelines that can help to maximize your nutrient intake and ensure you optimize your health during all the stages of the menopause.

The foundation of your menopause diet

Understanding how to balance macronutrients – proteins, fats, and carbohydrates (see pp.24–35) – efficiently is key to making sure you are getting the correct proportions of nutrients your body needs to function well. The panel, right, shows the ideal plate for the menopause. Getting adequate protein is essential now – it should be included in each meal (see pp.24–27). Generally women need to increase their protein intake in midlife to support health. Healthy fats (see pp.28–31) should be eaten regularly as these support hormone production and lower inflammation. You should eat a range of complex carbohydrates (see pp.32–35).

A range of nutrients

Micronutrients – vitamins and minerals – play a role in facilitating the production of hormones and other metabolic pathways, and help to limit damaging inflammation. A varied diet helps you meet your micronutrient needs. To get a good range of nutrients, vary ingredients

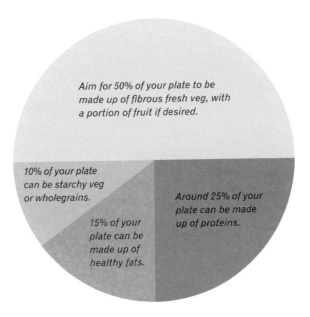

Aim for 50% of your plate to be made up of fibrous fresh veg, with a portion of fruit if desired.

10% of your plate can be starchy veg or wholegrains.

Around 25% of your plate can be made up of proteins.

15% of your plate can be made up of healthy fats.

The ideal plate

Follow the proportions of proteins, fats, and carbohydrates (in the form of vegetables and wholegrains) shown above to ensure you are getting a balanced diet.

regularly, including a single ingredient no more than three times a week. In addition, always try to alter food combinations, as certain nutrients compete for absorption so varying dishes helps to avoid insufficiencies.

Staying hydrated

Hydration is the basis of nutrition. Often, we are inadequately hydrated. Drinking 1.5 litres (2³/₄ pints) of water throughout the day gives us more energy, healthier skin, and improves digestion. Drink a glass of still water on waking, a glass with each meal or snack, and sip on a bottle between meals. If you wish, add pieces of lemon, lime, strawberry, blueberry, or cucumber, or fresh herbs, such as mint, rosemary, or sage. Foods with a high water content such as cucumber or courgette also hydrate. Limit mildly diuretic coffee and tea and avoid fizzy drinks and alcohol.

Eat more protein

Our bodies contain thousands of proteins, each with a specific function. Protein is vital for muscle and bone health and for regulating our immune system, but we often underestimate the importance of eating the right amount of protein. Furthermore, studies now suggest that as we reach the menopause, we need to up our protein intake.

How protein supports the menopause

Women approaching midlife are advised to increase their protein intake to 1–1.2 grams per kilogram of body weight per day, which for an average-sized woman equates to 20–25 grams with each meal.

Alongside regular exercise, protein helps to build muscle and maintain healthy bones. We reach peak bone density in our twenties and peak muscle mass in our thirties. Muscles then lose 3–5 per cent of their mass with each decade. Without sufficient protein from our diet, our bodies start to break down muscles to find the amino acids they need to build new proteins, which leads to further muscle wasting and an increased fracture risk from falls. Bone density also declines markedly post-menopause. Eating sufficient protein in midlife is vital for bone and muscle health in later years.

Protein, together with fats, also helps to regulate blood sugar levels, preventing the sugar highs and crashes that can exacerbate the menopausal fatigue caused by hormonal fluctuations and insomnia. Including protein in each meal also helps you to feel sated. This is because protein is made up of complex molecules, so it keeps you full for longer than simpler carbohydrates, removing the need to snack and in turn helping to curb menopausal weight gain.

Protein also helps to regulate the immune system, which is key to good health as we age.

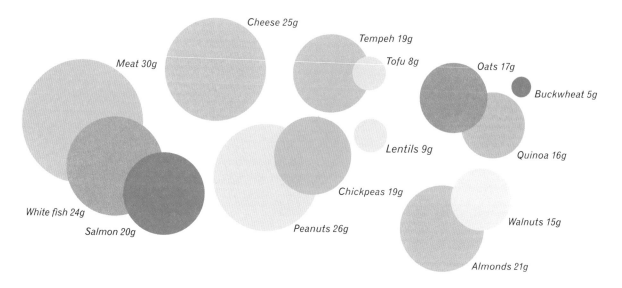

Cheese 25g

Tempeh 19g

Tofu 8g

Oats 17g

Meat 30g

Buckwheat 5g

Lentils 9g

Quinoa 16g

Chickpeas 19g

White fish 24g

Walnuts 15g

Salmon 20g

Peanuts 26g

Almonds 21g

Protein per 100g in key food groups

Most foods contain protein, but in different proportions. Per 100g, meats tend to have the highest amount of protein, followed by fish and seafood, cheese, nuts, and grains.

Types of protein

Our bodies need the building blocks known as amino acids that protein is made up of, so all protein is good for us. However, not all proteins are created equal. Of the 20 amino acids commonly found in plants and animals, there are two types: non-essential amino acids, which can be produced by the body as well as obtained from food, and essential amino acids, of which there are nine, which cannot be produced by the body and so must be obtained from our diet.

The proteins in animal-based foods such as meat, fish, eggs, and dairy are called complete proteins because they contain all nine essential amino acids. Most plant foods have incomplete proteins, which either lack some essential amino acids or provide them in insufficient quantities. If you are vegan or vegetarian, eating a variety of plant protein from grains, pulses, nuts, and seeds throughout the day will ensure you get the right amount of essential amino acids when caloric requirements are met.

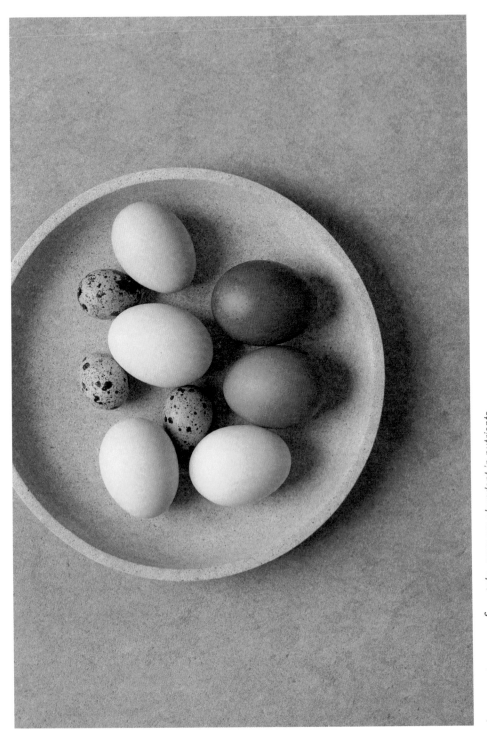

A compact source of protein, *eggs are abundant in nutrients.*

Complete proteins

Red meat, such as beef and lamb, and poultry, are not only the most protein-dense foods we can eat, they also have many other benefits. Opt for organic whenever possible, which has higher levels of omega-3 fats (see p.30). As well as protein, meat provides iron, selenium, and zinc, to boost immunity, and is high in B vitamins. The B vitamin family supports brain and heart health and helps our bodies cope with stress, but levels are often low in the menopause. Animal organs, such as liver, kidneys, brain, and tripe, are richest in nutrients. Poultry supplies an amino acid tryptophan, a precursor to serotonin, to lift the spirits and support sleep.

Fish and seafood are excellent sources of protein. Fish also has iodine, to support thyroid health, and oily fish are a top source of essential omega-3s and vitamin D. In addition, shellfish are densely packed with micronutrients such as selenium, zinc, iodine, iron, copper, and B12.

Eggs and dairy are fantastically versatile sources of animal protein. Chicken eggs are most popular, but other eggs such as quail, opposite, are equally nutritious. Eggs, impressively, boast an almost full quota of vitamins, excepting vitamin C. In addition, cholesterol in eggs aids the production of hormones such as oestrogen and testosterone. Dairy is a key source of calcium and vitamin D, both vital for bone health.

Soya products such as tofu, as well as the pseudograins buckwheat and quinoa, are plant proteins that contain all nine essential amino acids. Soya contains phytoestrogens (see p.44), so may also ease hot flushes.

Incomplete proteins

Plant sources of incomplete proteins include grains, as well as pulses such as chickpeas and lentils; beans; and nuts and seeds. Grains and pulses provide fibre and B vitamins, linked to a reduced risk of heart disease, while nuts and seeds are high in vitamin E, zinc, and calcium.

Choose the right fats

Fats – or lipids – are an essential component of a healthy diet. Although fat is the most calorific of all the nutrients, the body needs fat just as much as protein and carbohydrate. Polyunsaturated, monounsaturated, and saturated fats have a variety of important roles, enabling the body to absorb fat-soluble vitamins, providing energy, supporting cognition, and producing hormones, all vital for health throughout the menopause.

How fats support the menopause

Including sources of fat at each meal delivers a wide range of benefits. Aim for about 15 per cent of your plate to comprise a healthy fat, such as a tablespoon of olive oil or a portion of oily fish. Fats are an important source of energy, which is often chronically low in the menopause. They also contribute to our sense of fullness. This is because the process of breaking down fatty foods in the digestive system is a lengthy one so this promotes a lasting feeling of being full. Feeling satiated helps to reduce cravings for unhealthy snacks, so including fats as part of an overall healthy diet is an important part of controlling midlife weight gain.

Saturated fats help the body produce sex hormones. A healthy amount of fat also plays a protective role for organs such as the heart, kidneys, and liver, cushioning and protecting them.

Fats are key to digestion. Without fats, the body is unable to absorb certain key nutrients, such as the fat-soluble vitamins A, D, E, and K; lycopene (obtained from tomatoes); and antioxidant betacarotene (found in colourful fruits and vegetables such as carrots).

The role of cholesterol

Cholesterol is a substance present in animal fats and is also produced by our livers. Cholesterol plays a vital role in our bodies.

While too high levels of cholesterol in the blood are associated with artery disease, cholesterol is vital for our bodies. It is an essential component of our cell membranes that is beneficial for brain health, nerves, and skin. Cholesterol also helps our bodies to make bile, which is needed to digest fats, in turn helping to control weight. It is involved in the production of vitamin D, which is hard to source from food yet is essential for bone health. Cholesterol also plays a part in the production of steroid hormones, including cortisol, testosterone, progesterone, and oestrogen, which help to keep our bones, teeth, and muscles strong and healthy.

Types of fat

The lipids, or fat, family is the most complex of the three macronutrients – fats, proteins, and carbohydrates. A healthy diet includes a combination of polyunsaturated, monounsaturated, and saturated fats (which are solid at room temperature). Another fat – trans fat – is formed through a process of hydrogenation and is found in some processed foods, such as crisps and pies, and this should always be avoided (see p.51).

Continued studies on the effects of fats have led to evolving opinions on certain types of fat. Science recognizes that polyunsaturated omega-3 fats and monounsaturated fats have significant health benefits and lower levels of bad cholesterol in the body. Saturated fat has often been discussed as a fat to avoid and linked to an increased risk of conditions such as heart disease. However, recent research has led to the consensus on good and bad fats shifting. It is now thought that it is what you eat with saturated fats – such as sugary, processed foods – that may raise your risk of cardiovascular disease more than the actual fat itself.

Saturated fats

Found mainly in animal products and in some plant foods such as coconut and palm oil, these help to produce hormones. Foods with saturated fat often have a range of health benefits. For example, grass-fed beef provides antioxidants and polyunsaturated omega-3s; dairy provides minerals and vitamin D for bones; and live yogurt and kefir have probiotics to boost healthy gut bacteria. Recent research suggests that coconut oil may raise good cholesterol and support cognition.

Polyunsaturated fats

Oily fish, such as salmon, mackerel, anchovies, sardines, and fresh tuna, are top sources of polyunsaturated omega-3 fats, which are crucial for our health. Omega-3s have a range of powerful benefits, from supporting heart and brain health and strengthening our immunity to promoting deep sleep. They are especially helpful for symptoms such as hot flushes, low mood, and joint pain. Flax, pumpkin and hemp seeds, and walnuts also supply omega-3.

Omega-6, also vital, is found in poultry, nuts, cereals, and vegetable oils. Our bodies need more omega-3 than omega-6. However, because omega-6 is more easily found in foods, the ratio of omega-6 to omega-3 in our bodies is often less than ideal, so upping our intake of omega-3 sources would be beneficial.

Monounsaturated fats

Found in avocados and olives, nut-based oils, and in nuts and seeds, these play a significant role in maintaining our cardiovascular health.

Avocado is a compact source of key nutrients, including vitamin K, folate, and vitamin C, as well as potassium. Most avocado fat is a fatty acid called oleic acid, which is thought to promote healthy blood pressure. Avocados are also a great source of fibre, easing digestion and reducing sugar spikes and the subsequent energy dips.

Olives and olive oils are also high in oleic acid and are very high in skin-nourishing vitamin E, promoting healthy looking skin as you age.

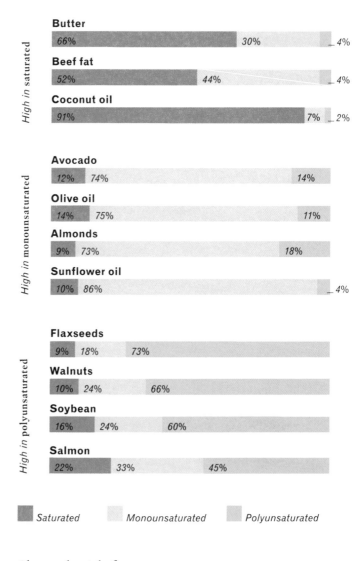

High in saturated

Butter
66% | 30% | 4%

Beef fat
52% | 44% | 4%

Coconut oil
91% | 7% | 2%

High in monounsaturated

Avocado
12% | 74% | 14%

Olive oil
14% | 75% | 11%

Almonds
9% | 73% | 18%

Sunflower oil
10% | 86% | 4%

High in polyunsaturated

Flaxseeds
9% | 18% | 73%

Walnuts
10% | 24% | 66%

Soybean
16% | 24% | 60%

Salmon
22% | 33% | 45%

■ *Saturated*   *Monounsaturated*   *Polyunsaturated*

Choose the right fats

*All foods that contain fat have a variety of saturated,
monounsaturated, and polyunsaturated fatty acids,
with some especially high in a particular type of fat.*

Rethink carbohydrates

Unrefined, complex carbohydrates (see p.35) are an essential part of a healthy diet and may also help to ease certain menopausal symptoms. They may help to control blood sugar levels, avoiding energy slumps, and are also an important source of fibre to support digestion. Carbohydrates should make up the majority of our daily food intake, so it is important to understand how to make them work for you.

How carbohydrates support the menopause

Carbohydrates are broken down into glucose relatively quickly, so they have a more pronounced effect on blood sugar levels than either fat or protein. Eating carbohydrates with proteins and fats and choosing complex rather than simple carbohydrates will have the least impact on your blood sugar levels. During the menopause, steady blood sugar levels help to keep energy levels constant, in turn helping to stabilize moods and control weight gain as the desire to snack on sugary, unhealthy foods is diminished. The glycaemic index (GI) (see opposite) rates carbohydrates in different foods by how quickly each food affects our blood sugar levels.

Complex carbohydrates are also an important source of dietary fibre, both soluble and insoluble, helping to optimize digestion. Plant foods have varying proportions of soluble fibre – which absorbs water, breaking down to help reduce blood sugar spikes – and insoluble fibre – which does not break down, but acts as a bulking agent to speed the passage of waste through the gut. Eating plenty of fibre – while also maintaining an adequate water intake to help fibre move smoothly through the digestive tract – helps to relieve common menopausal complaints such as constipation.

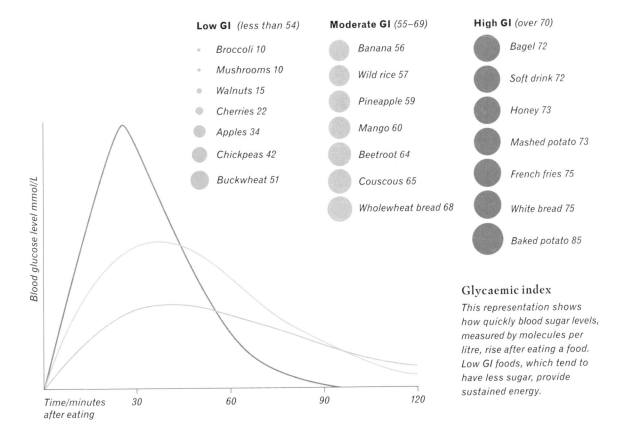

Low GI *(less than 54)*

- Broccoli 10
- Mushrooms 10
- Walnuts 15
- Cherries 22
- Apples 34
- Chickpeas 42
- Buckwheat 51

Moderate GI *(55–69)*

- Banana 56
- Wild rice 57
- Pineapple 59
- Mango 60
- Beetroot 64
- Couscous 65
- Wholewheat bread 68

High GI *(over 70)*

- Bagel 72
- Soft drink 72
- Honey 73
- Mashed potato 73
- French fries 75
- White bread 75
- Baked potato 85

Blood glucose level mmol/L

Time/minutes after eating

30   60   90   120

Glycaemic index

This representation shows how quickly blood sugar levels, measured by molecules per litre, rise after eating a food. Low GI foods, which tend to have less sugar, provide sustained energy.

Some soluble fibres are called fermentable fibres, which means that our gut bacteria can digest these fibres. By increasing and balancing friendly gut bacteria, these soluble fibres help to maintain our gut and metabolic health.

Many complex carbohydrates are also naturally high in essential vitamins, minerals, and phytonutrients – the natural compounds, such as flavonoids, carotenoids, glucosinolates, and resveratrol, that are produced by plants to protect them from external threats. Making sure that your diet is rich in phytonutrients reaps rewards as you will benefit from their antioxidant and anti-inflammatory properties (see pp.36–39). Controlling inflammation is crucial during midlife and beyond as this promotes healthy brain function and protects the body against cardiovascular disease.

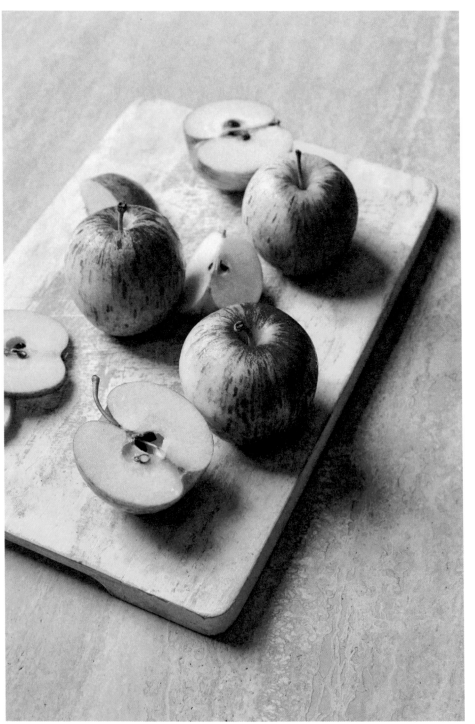

Apples provide essential fibre for a healthy menopause diet.

Types of carbohydrate

There are two types of carbohydrate: simple and complex. Simple carbohydrates, also called sugars, are found in refined foods such as biscuits, sugary cereals, pasta, and white bread. Broken down quickly by the body, these raise blood sugar levels rapidly, causing energy spikes and slumps, and so are best avoided.

Complex carbohydrates are found in fruits and vegetables, wholegrains, legumes, pulses, and nuts and seeds. They contain starches and fibre, which are broken down more slowly, raising sugar levels steadily.

Complex carbohydrates

Wholegrains (see pp.40–43) are complex high-fibre carbohydrates that support bowel function, so they can play an extremely helpful role in the menopause by easing uncomfortable constipation. They also help us manage our weight, which not only helps us to feel confident in the menopause, but also reduces the risk of conditions such as diabetes. Furthermore, wholegrains supply proteins, B vitamins – crucial for managing stress (see p.40) – and a host of antioxidant minerals.

Legumes and pulses are unrefined complex carbohydrates that are high in vitamin E, zinc, and calcium, helping to nourish thinning skin and support bone health. They also provide a compound called boron, which plays a key role in bone health, so is crucial in midlife.

Starchy vegetables and fruit such as beetroot, apples, bananas, squash, and sweet potatoes, as well as fibrous produce, such as broccoli, asparagus, radishes, and mushrooms (see pp.36–39), provide not only carbohydrates, but also micronutrients such as vitamin C and potassium.

Nuts and seeds (see also p.27) add some carbohydrates, as well as fibre and protein to our diets, helping to regulate blood sugar and aid digestion.

Increase your vegetable and fruit intake

Ensuring that you regularly eat a wide range of vegetables as well as some fresh fruit is a crucial part of a healthy menopause diet, providing a variety of vitamins, minerals, and phytonutrients, key for overall health, as well as fibre (see p.32), to aid digestion.

How vegetables and fruit support the menopause

Eating a "rainbow" of different-coloured vegetables and fruit ensures that your body receives a range of phytonutrients (see p.39) that have protective antioxidant and anti-inflammatory properties. Flavonoids, one of the largest groups of phytonutrients, and resveratrol, protect against cardiovascular disease, an increased risk as oestrogen falls. Carotenoids, found in bright produce, support immune health, while glucosinolates, in cruciferous vegetables, promote cardiovascular and cognitive health.

Making vegetables and fruit a cornerstone of your diet also increases your intake of fibre, promoting healthy bowel function and in turn reducing unwelcome menopausal symptoms such as constipation and bloating, which can make us feel sluggish.

Vegetables and fruit play a vital role in maintaining a healthy, diverse gut microbiome – the collection of microorganisms in the form of bacteria, viruses, protozoa, and fungi that inhabit the gastrointestinal tract. A healthy gut microbiome is key for immunity and also helps reduce inflammation, protecting against disease in midlife. Fermented vegetables such as sauerkraut and kimchi and pickled vegetables provide probiotics – the live "good" bacteria that populate our guts. A whole range of fruit and vegetables, such as unripe bananas, onions, leeks, garlic, and asparagus, provide prebiotics – the plant fibres that feed probiotics, boosting the existing friendly bacteria in our guts.

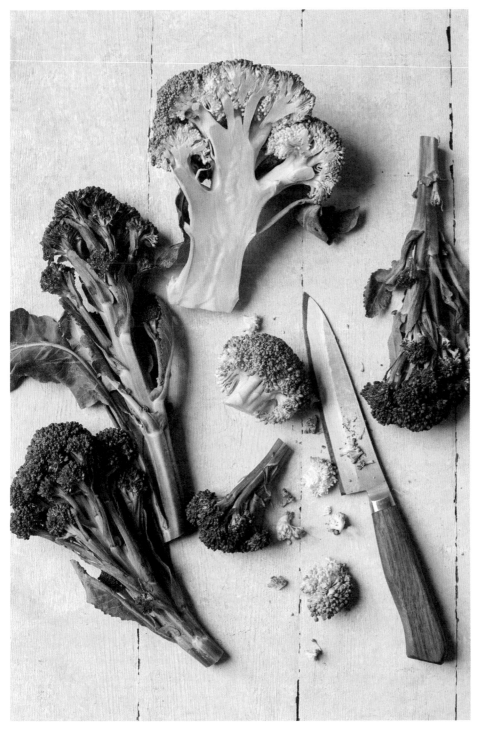

Broccoli, a key source of phytonutrients, *has anti-inflammatory properties.*

Cruciferous vegetables

Also called brassicas, cruciferous vegetables are key in the menopause. They include broccoli, cauliflower, kale, watercress, and rocket, as well as bok choy, cabbage, kohlrabi, and radishes. Brassicas have a compound called indole-3-carbinol (I3C), which is broken down by stomach acids to form a compound called diindolylmethane (DIM). This in turn helps balance oestrogen, may protect against some cancers, and stimulates fat breakdown.

Individual brassicas also have particular benefits. For instance, broccoli has a potent antioxidant sulforaphane and the flavonoid kaempferol, both anti-inflammatories, while cauliflower is high in antioxidants such as glucosinolates, carotenoids, and flavonoids, which support cardiovascular health, as well as immune-boosting vitamin C. Watercress, incredibly, has 40 unique flavonoids, protecting cells from damage and lowering the risk of diabetes and heart disease. Radishes have the cancer-fighting antioxidant compound indole-3-carbinol.

Leafy greens

Greens such as spinach and kale are packed with antioxidants. Spinach provides nitrates, which promote healthy blood vessels, as well as anti-inflammatory quercetin. Kale has betacarotene, vitamin C, necessary for the synthesis of skin-plumping collagen, flavonoids, and polyphenols, which support heart health and help lift mood.

Root vegetables

These high-fibre vegetables have an abundance of benefits. Beetroot provides iron, manganese, potassium, and vitamin C, while carrots and sweet potatoes have betacarotene, to support cognition and memory.

Other vegetables

Bright produce such as squash, tomatoes, and peppers are an important source of immune-boosting vitamin C, while meaty mushrooms contain polysaccharide beta glucans, which are thought to raise levels of good cholesterol in the body. Asparagus supplies vitamin E for skin health, immune-boosting vitamin C, and heart-protecting polyphenols. Include vegetables with a high water content, such as courgettes and cucumbers, in your diet regularly to keep the body well hydrated.

Green produce

- broccoli
- leafy greens
- cruciferous veg
- green peppers
- peas
- courgettes

Green-coloured produce is high in chlorophyll, glucosinolates, vitamin K, and carotenoids for bone and heart health.

Bright produce

- oranges
- peppers
- squash
- citrus fruit
- beetroot
- apricots
- bananas
- sweet potato

Orange and yellow produce is especially high in betacarotene and vitamins A and C, for heart health and immunity; red produce provides flavonoids, lycopene, and vitamin C, for cognition and heart health.

Purple/blue produce

- berries
- aubergines
- grapes
- peppers

Purple and blue-hued fruit and vegetables are especially high in anthocyanin, which promotes cognitive health and protects against the effects of ageing.

Eating a rainbow of produce

Eating a variety of different-coloured vegetables and fruit ensures that you receive a wide range of therapeutic antioxidant phytonutrients.

In addition, making the allium family – onions, garlic, leeks, and spring onions – the basis of meals promotes gut health, reduces inflammation, and aids cognition.

Fruits

Sweet or tangy, and always delicious, antioxidant-rich fruits have a range of benefits for the menopause. Enjoy antioxidant-rich berries to support healthy blood pressure; vitamin C-rich citrus and tropical fruits for immunity, skin, and blood vessel health; and apples for bone-supporting boron.

Opt for wholegrains

Grains are small, hard, edible dry seeds that grow on grass-like cereal plants and are an important source of energy. Wholegrains are made up of all the essential parts of the grain, so contain the naturally occurring nutrients of the entire grain seed in their original proportions. In contrast, highly processed refined grains such as white flour have had some nutrients removed.

How wholegrains support the menopause

Wholegrains are a valuable part of a healthy and balanced menopause diet. Whether cracked, crushed, rolled, or cooked, they retain the nutrient-dense outer layer of the grain called the bran, making them an excellent source of dietary fibre. As well as supporting digestion, wholegrains are low in sugar, so don't cause blood sugar levels to spike, which in turn provides steady energy. They are also beneficial for gut bacteria. It is important to cook wholegrains properly so they are digested efficiently.

Wholegrains are a rich source of nutrients. They provide many B vitamins, which are crucial during the menopause. B vitamins help the body to metabolize fats, proteins, and carbohydrates to provide energy, and are also vital for the healthy functioning of the nervous system, both of which makes them important for managing stress. Furthermore, if vitamins B6, B9, and B12 are deficient, this can contribute to a number of conditions such as anaemia, depression, and memory loss, so it is vital to ensure that you include good sources regularly in your diet.

Wholegrains also provide essential minerals, including phosphorous, manganese, and selenium, which occur in varying amounts in different grains. Phosphorous and manganese are both essential for healthy bones, helping to maintain mineral bone density in midlife and so reduce the likelihood of osteoporosis developing post-menopause,

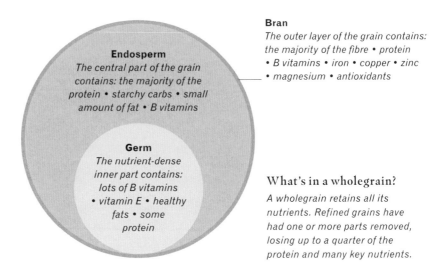

Endosperm
The central part of the grain contains: the majority of the protein • starchy carbs • small amount of fat • B vitamins

Bran
The outer layer of the grain contains: the majority of the fibre • protein • B vitamins • iron • copper • zinc • magnesium • antioxidants

Germ
The nutrient-dense inner part contains: lots of B vitamins • vitamin E • healthy fats • some protein

What's in a wholegrain?
A wholegrain retains all its nutrients. Refined grains have had one or more parts removed, losing up to a quarter of the protein and many key nutrients.

when the ovaries stop producing protective oestrogen. Manganese also supports brain and nerve function and is involved in the metabolism of fats and carbohydrates. And selenium is an important antioxidant whose anti-inflammatory properties help to promote healthy cognition in the menopause as well as support a robust immune system.

Gluten and the menopause

Gluten, a protein found in wheat, barley, and rye, can be problematic for many women, who often are unaware that their symptoms may be linked to a gluten sensitivity. While the autoimmune disorder coeliac disease is well documented, less well understood is non-coeliac gluten sensitivity, which is linked to over 100 conditions, many of which are common in the menopause, so may be overlooked as hormone-related.

Gluten sensitivity can worsen or develop during the menopause, causing inflammation, so avoiding or reducing gluten may ease symptoms. Menopause makes the digestive system less efficient at breaking down foods, which means that larger, undigested particles can escape and trigger the immune system, leading to a reaction. Signs of gluten intolerance include bloating, cramping, constipation and/or diarrhoea, excess gas, and mental symptoms such as brain fog, depression, and fatigue.

Going gluten-free

Gluten-free sections in supermarkets often have processed foods with poor-quality ingredients. The best way to transition is to cook and bake with naturally gluten-free grains and, whenever possible, avoid gluten-free processed foods. Gluten-free grains do lack the elasticity of gluten, but there are some excellent flours available (see below).

Naturally gluten-free grains

There are lots of nutritious gluten-free grains to choose from. Try quinoa, buckwheat (pseudograins, that is, seeds with some grain characteristics), all types of rice, and oats, all used in the recipes in this book, as well as amaranth, corn, millet, or sorghum. Bear in mind that while oats are gluten-free, they are often processed in factories with gluten-containing grains so can be contaminated. Look for oats labelled gluten-free to be sure.

Buckwheat has impressive benefits. It is made into nuggety granules, or groats, which can be ground down into flour to use in baking and bread. A source of protein and fibre, buckwheat also has phytonutrients and the key minerals magnesium and manganese. A polyphenol rutin in buckwheat has anti-inflammatory properties that may help to lower the risk of heart disease. It is thought to support blood flow, promoting healthy blood pressure. Buckwheat also contains quercetin, from the group of anti-inflammatory phytonutrient flavonoids, while a molecule called D-chiro-inositol in buckwheat helps to reduce blood sugars, lowering the risk of diabetes.

Quinoa is nutrient-dense and a valuable addition to a menopause diet. It contains the anti-inflammatory, anti-viral, and mood-lifting flavonoid kaempferol.

Rice and wild rice contain a range of anti-inflammatory antioxidants, including flavonoids, all of which promote heart health. Though filling, its low calorie content makes it a great choice for weight control.

Oats support cardiovascular health, which is affected by oestrogen decline, and are high in the amino acid tryptophan, involved in serotonin production, helping to lift mood and promote restful sleep.

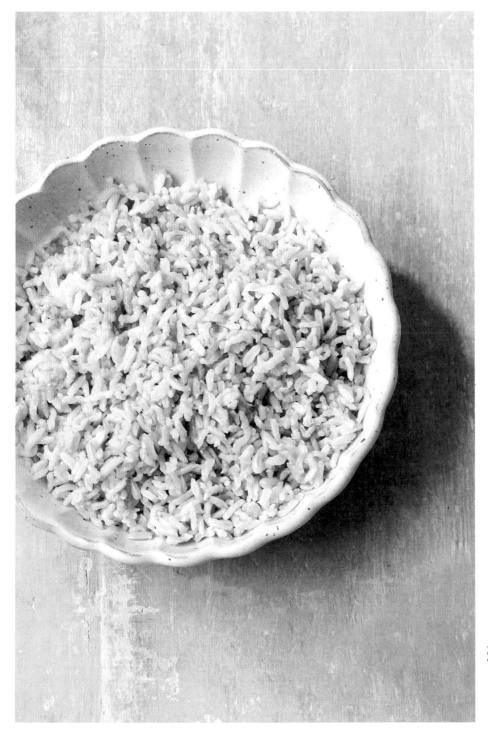

A source of fibre, rice helps sate the appetite and control weight gain.

Opt for wholegrains

Find phytoestrogens

Phytoestrogens are natural chemicals or compounds produced by plants that have a similar chemical structure to the oestrogen produced in our bodies. When we consume phytoestrogens, they interact weakly with human oestrogen receptors, making the body believe that it has more oestrogen than it does. Phytoestrogens are commonly associated with soy food products, but they are also found in a number of other foods (see opposite and p.47). Including phytoestrogens in your diet as you approach midlife and throughout the menopause years may help to reduce the severity of some common menopausal symptoms.

How phytoestrogens support the menopause

Phytoestrogens are weaker than natural oestrogens, but studies show that a higher dietary intake of them can help ease some common menopausal symptoms. There is no recommended daily amount of phytoestrogens, but you can include them regularly in your diet.

Phytoestrogens are thought to be most effective in helping to ease hot flushes and night sweats, relieving the physical discomfort and anxiety that these symptoms cause and resulting in a better quality of life. A group of phytoestrogens called isoflavones (see below and opposite) are thought to promote artery health as well as support bone health, protecting against osteoporosis post-menopause.

Types of phytoestrogens

There are several classes of phytoestrogens but the two best-known groups of these compounds are isoflavones and lignans. Isoflavones are a group of molecules that are found in soy products and legumes, such

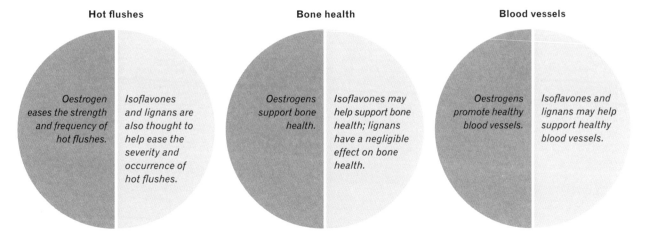

Hot flushes

Oestrogen eases the strength and frequency of hot flushes.

Isoflavones and lignans are also thought to help ease the severity and occurrence of hot flushes.

Bone health

Oestrogens support bone health.

Isoflavones may help support bone health; lignans have a negligible effect on bone health.

Blood vessels

Oestrogens promote healthy blood vessels.

Isoflavones and lignans may help support healthy blood vessels.

How isoflavones and lignans help with symptoms

The action of isoflavones and lignans is similar to oestrogen. Though their effects are more limited, they are helpful for easing vasomotor symptoms such as hot flushes.

as chickpeas, mung beans, lentils, beans, and alfalfa. Lignans are found in flaxseeds, sunflower seeds, wheat, oats, barley, and rice.

Soy-based foods

Processed soybeans form the basis of an assortment of plant-based food products, including tempeh, tofu, and miso. Unprocessed, raw soybeans are called edamame. Both soybeans and edamame are high in isoflavones. These are one of the most potent phytoestrogens, helping to reduce uncomfortable vasomotor symptoms such as hot flushes and night sweats. The isoflavones in soybeans need to be broken down into four compounds and converted by the gut into oestrogenic substances, which can make it hard for the body to access them. To help the body metabolize isoflavones, opt for fermented soy products such as miso and tempeh and avoid highly processed soy products such as soy milk, soy yogurt, and soy desserts.

Tofu, tempeh, and miso all help to ease hot flushes. Tofu has benefits for heart, bone, and brain health and helps balance blood sugars, reducing the risk of diabetes. It is also a filling protein, helping to

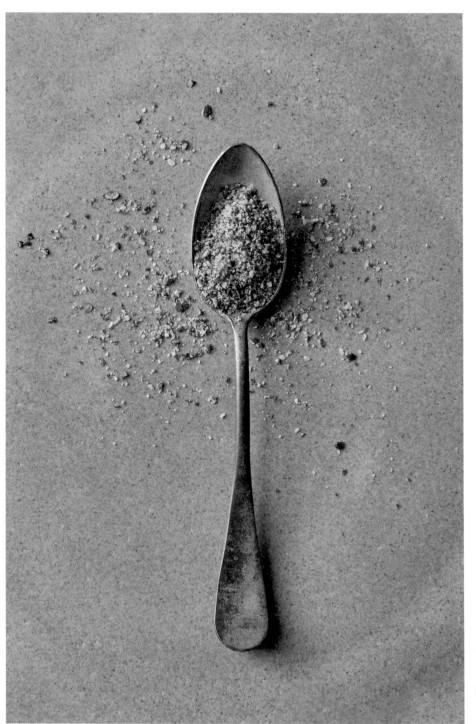

Tiny flaxseeds *have an impressive nutrient profile.*

manage weight gain. Miso supports heart and brain health. Both miso and tempeh act as probiotics (see p.36).

Seeds, nuts, and grains

Easy to add to dishes or simply enjoyed as a snack, flaxseeds (shown opposite) and sesame seeds are valuable phytoestrogens. They contain lignans, which may ease symptoms such as hot flushes. Both seeds contain heart-supporting omega-3s; flaxseeds also help to control blood sugar levels, avoiding energy slumps that can exacerbate menopausal fatigue. Sesame seeds have anti-inflammatory properties and contain calcium and magnesium, both supportive of bone health.

Rice, oats, quinoa, barley, rye, and wheat bran also have concentrated amounts of beneficial lignans.

Legumes

Chickpeas, lentils, red kidney beans, and split peas are high in isoflavones. While all nutritious, chickpeas are an especially good choice for vegetarians and vegans in the menopause. As well as being phytoestrogenic, they are a good plant source of protein.

Fruit and vegetables

Alongside their anti-inflammatory properties, cruciferous vegetables are a rich source of phytoestrogens. Summer berries, such as raspberries and strawberries, also provide phytoestrogens, as well as being densely packed with phytonutrients and a source of digestion-supporting fibre.

Sprouted seeds

Sprouted seeds, such as alfalfa, mung bean, and broccoli sprouts, are a prime source of phytoestrogens. Sprouting seeds is a fantastic and easy way to increase your intake of macro- and micronutrients, boosting levels of protein, folate, magnesium, phosphorus, manganese, vitamins C and K, and natural enzymes.

Sprouted seeds are easy to digest, helping to relieve complaints such as constipation and bloating. Broccoli, radish, cress, and clover sprouts are especially helpful for relieving menopausal hot flushes.

Supplements in the menopause

A plethora of menopause supplements on the market can leave women feeling that they should supplement their diets as a matter of course. Ideally, it is always best to optimize your diet and lifestyle to avoid the need for supplements. If you do feel that a supplement would be helpful, consult a qualified nutritionist who can recommend specific supplements tailored to your symptoms. Bear in mind, too, that supplements are intended to address temporary shortfalls rather than be a long-term solution.

Why we might need supplements

A number of contributing factors can mean that supplementing your diet is sometimes helpful in the menopause. Generally, the growth in intensive farming, with monocrop soil lacking in minerals and fruits harvested for shipping before they are ripe, can impact the nutrients available in fresh produce.

This can be compounded by the fact that many of us could improve our diets, which are often lacking in certain nutrients. In addition, chronic stress from busy lives, an increase in medication as we get older, which can interfere with the body's ability to absorb nutrients, and pollution all mean that it can be easy to enter the menopause with a below par nutrient pool. Good nutrition is key for coping with the demands of the menopause. In addition, being low in key nutrients in midlife makes it easier to develop menopausal symptoms and conditions that will make the menopause transition harder. Supplementing the diet can help fill some nutritional gaps.

Supplements for the menopause

A multivitamin and mineral supplement for women aged over 40 can be beneficial, in addition to improving diet and lifestyle. Nutrients that are especially helpful include magnesium for heart health, digestion, sleep, anxiety, cognition, and muscles; vitamins D3 and K2 for bone health; and omega-3 supplements (EPA and DHA) for cardiovascular health.

It is always best to consult a medical practitioner before taking supplements. They can assess which ones you need, and guide you on dosage, when and how to take a supplement, and for how long.

As well as commercial supplements, culinary herbs and spices have specific properties that can be used as natural supplements.

- **Sage** may ease hot flushes and night sweats and aid cognition.
- **Rosemary** has a soothing effect on nerves, pain, indigestion, and allergies, and its aroma has been shown to boost memory.
- **Thyme** supports healthy blood pressure, cholesterol, and immunity.
- **Parsley, basil, and turmeric** have anti-inflammatory properties for joint and cardiovascular health and parsley aids digestion.
- **Mint and peppermint** ease nausea and aid digestion.
- **Cinnamon** promotes healthy blood sugar levels.
- **Ginger** eases nausea and stimulates blood supply.

What to avoid

Nutrition is not just about including the right foods in your diet, it is also about removing foods and drinks that can be harmful and contribute to weight gain. Certain foods also act as trigger foods, causing or exacerbating menopause symptoms, so removing these from your diet and finding alternatives can have excellent results. Many of the foods below have been shown to have an impact on specific menopause symptoms, as well as on general health.

The impact of a poor diet in the menopause

The menopause transition can be challenging, with symptoms such as easier weight gain leading to discomfort and increasing health risks. An unhealthy diet exacerbates symptoms, making it harder to lose weight and increasing the risk of conditions such as diabetes. Making long-term changes to address unhealthy lifestyle habits now will help your body to heal and make weight loss easier.

Eliminating dietary triggers

Certain foods and drinks have been shown to have a detrimental impact on menopausal symptoms. By eliminating them and finding healthier alternatives whenever possible, you may find your menopause symptoms are reduced.

- **Hot, spicy foods** contain the compound capsaicin, which has a dilating effect on blood vessels that can trigger sweating and hot flushes. If you suffer with hot flushes, avoid spices or opt for milder ones, such as turmeric, cumin, and mild curry powder, which are packed with flavour but have less heat.

- **Caffeine**, especially in coffee, can also increase the risk of hot flushes and often impacts sleep quality. Try to limit your coffee intake to one cup a day, as early in the morning as possible. Try swapping coffee for herbal teas or green tea, which has less caffeine, and opt for water throughout the day to help reduce your caffeine intake.
- **Hot drinks** are thought to trigger hot flushes in some women. If this is the case, swap them for lukewarm or cold drinks. Cold drinks can also actively relieve hot flushes.
- **Alcohol** can aggravate hot flushes and also impacts on quality of sleep. Taking a break from alcohol or reducing your consumption can benefit your health. If you think there is a link between your consumption and hot flushes, you could also try recording what you drink (the type of wine, beer, or spirit), how much, and how long after drinking you experience a hot flush, detailing its severity and duration, to see if there is a link with a particular drink.
- **Sugary foods**, which are often processed foods, not only trigger cravings and make weight gain more likely, but they also increase your risk of developing conditions such as diabetes, cholesterol, and cardiovascular disease, which menopausal and post-menopausal women are more vulnerable to.
- **Trans fats**, or trans fatty acids, are formed through a process of hydrogenation, where adding hydrogen atoms turns oils into solid fats. The health risks posed by trans fats are well documented. They have been linked to an increase in unhealthy cholesterol levels, heart disease, inflammation, stroke, diabetes, and other chronic health conditions, so should be avoided at all costs. Trans fats are found in small quantities in animal foods, but most come from processed foods. These harmful fats are being phased out, however it is still possible to find them in some margarines, shortening, and other processed foods, where they are labelled as hydrogenated or partially hydrogenated fats. While ready-meals and processed foods can seem convenient, they can have profound effects on long-term health.

Looking at lifestyle

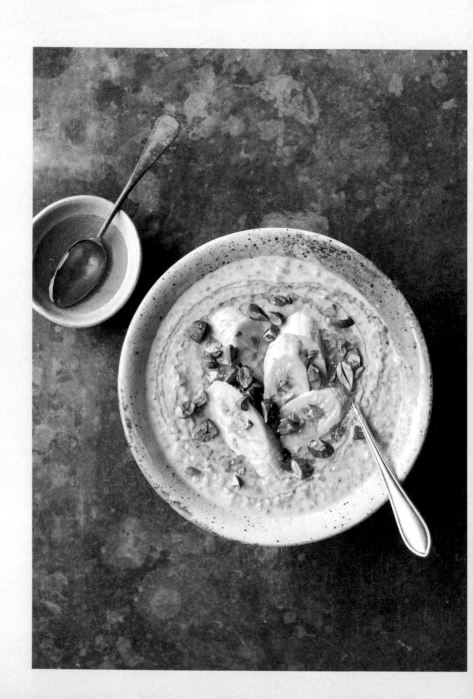

Your diet is just one, albeit extremely important, element of staying healthy during the menopause. To enjoy optimal health throughout this time of change, you need to take a holistic approach to your lifestyle and make sure that enjoying a healthy diet is married with a whole lifestyle check.

The mental and physical challenges that the menopause years can present mean you need to equip each aspect of your life to cope. Your quality of sleep, the levels of activity you undertake, and the ways in which you cope with everyday stressors are all interwoven – managing one of these areas can have a beneficial and often lasting impact on the others. The following chapter explores ways to help you enjoy restful and restorative sleep; offers an overview on how you can maintain fitness or gradually build your levels of activity; and looks at simple ways to cope with and minimize the impact of stress. In addition, it also helps you to understand the medication options as well as some of the natural therapies that are available to help you manage menopause symptoms, enabling you to build a complete set of strategies to cope and thrive in these menopause years.

Other lifestyle approaches

The menopause transition presents new challenges with symptoms such as anxiety and fatigue that can sometimes feel overwhelming. Addressing nutrition is the first step to optimizing health now, as once we are fully hydrated and nourished, we sleep better, feel more energized on waking, are less stressed, more focused, and enjoy better digestion. However, nutrition is only one of the four pillars of good health. Movement, sleep, and stress management are also key. In addition, you may want to consider the role of hormone replacement therapy (HRT) and natural remedies to help you cope in the menopause.

Taking a proactive approach

While we are aware that adopting an active lifestyle, getting sufficient good-quality sleep, and finding ways to manage everyday stress are fundamental to health and wellbeing, when we feel below par, we often neglect to focus actively on these areas. We may reassure ourselves that we will start to exercise again when our joints are less stiff. We may think there is nothing we can do about frequently waking in the night because this is to be expected in the menopause, or we may feel that the stress that is caused by menopause symptoms is inevitable.

However, giving each of these areas due attention – looking at how to stay active, improve sleep, and address stress – will reap benefits. The advice, tips, and guidelines on pages 56–61 will equip you with strategies to help manage these important areas, allowing you to enjoy a good quality of life throughout the menopause.

When extra help is needed

Sometimes natural approaches alone are not sufficient to improve menopausal symptoms, or you may feel you simply need some extra help to make your symptoms manageable. Bear in mind that symptoms can last for several years so finding what works for you early on will make your day-to-day life easier. Being informed about the options available and their pros and cons and following your instincts can help you decide on the best course of action.

Pages 62–63 look at the role of hormone replacement therapy (HRT) and other prescription medications and how these can help alongside lifestyle measures. You may also want to explore some of the complementary therapies discussed on pages 64–65, many of which have been shown to help with menopausal symptoms.

Ultimately, whether or not you take medication remains your own decision. Health practitioners can advise you, but you are the only person living in your body and experiencing your life.

Reducing lifestyle toxins

Trying to limit everyday toxins helps to optimize health in midlife. Our "toxic load" refers to the toxins and chemicals in our bodies that we ingest from various sources, including the air we breathe, the food we eat, the water we drink, and the personal care and household products we use. Many toxins contain chemicals called xenoestrogens, which are linked to cancer. Like the plant molecules, phytoestrogens, these bind to human oestrogen receptors, mimicking natural oestrogen compounds. These hormone disruptors are found in chemical compounds such as PCBs, BPAs, phthalates, and triclosan, and are linked to conditions such as migraines, breast problems, and thyroid imbalances. The chemicals are present in shampoos, body lotions, deodorants, toothpaste, and various household products. Checking ingredients helps to avoid these chemicals; online sources can show you which ingredients to look out for. Drinking filtered water and eating organic produce whenever possible will also help you to reduce your toxic load.

An active lifestyle

Movement and exercise keep us in shape physically and mentally. As we get older, it can be tempting to reduce our levels of activity, perhaps because of lack of time or pain or discomfort. However, the menopause is possibly the most important time to continue, or take up, physical activities.

Exercise and movement

Staying active allows us to function and remain independent. Building activity into your routine helps maintain a healthy cardiovascular system so that the body can carry nutrients to cells and remove toxins via the lymphatic system. The contraction of skeletal muscles also helps push blood and lymph around the body.

How staying active helps in the menopause

Making movement and exercise an integral part of your lifestyle has significant benefits during the menopause. Strength training and weight-bearing activities, such as walking, running, and tennis, help to slow the decline of bone mineral density, reducing the risk of sarcopenia (loss of muscle mass) and osteoporosis. Regular exercise also helps to manage weight; can reduce the severity of hot flushes; and supports sleep. In addition, being active helps us to remain mobile, reduces lower back pain and stress, and lifts depression. Even moderate physical activities that move the body enough to raise the heart rate a little, help to energize us and improve health. Ideally, exercise should be sufficient to raise your heart rate without making you out of breath or exhausted.

Find an activity that is manageable in the long term. Doing something that you enjoy will help to motivate you and make it more likely that you will continue. Recruiting an exercise buddy, depending on your personality, can also be a great motivator.

Building an exercise regime

If you already have an active lifestyle, continue with this. If you are sedentary, increase activity slowly, maybe starting by aiming to walk 10,000 steps a day. Once this feels easy, consider adding activities. Stretching exercises improve movement in your upper and lower body, then you can move on to more vigorous exercises if you wish.

The table below charts the benefits of different exercise types. An effective regime could be resistance and weight-bearing exercises three days a week on alternate days, then activities such as brisk walking, cycling, gardening, or dancing on the other days. Warm up first and talk to your healthcare practitioner before exercising if you suffer with conditions such as osteoporosis, heart problems, or severe stress.

Types of exercise and benefits	Examples
Cardiovascular *Strengthens the heart, respiration, and large muscle groups.*	*Running, jogging, cycling, swimming.*
Weight-bearing, high-impact *Maintains bone strength. Avoid with conditions such as osteoporosis or if you have persistent backache.*	*Dancing, high-impact aerobics, running, jogging, skipping, and stair climbing; sports such as tennis.*
Weight-bearing, low-impact *Helps to maintain bone strength; ideal for those who struggle with high-impact exercise.*	*Walking (on a treadmill or outside), elliptical training machines, stair-step machines, and low-impact aerobics.*
Weight, strength, or resistance training exercises *Builds strength and maintains muscle mass in midlife.*	*Lifting weights; using elastic bands or weight machines; simple movements such as standing or lifting own body weight.*
Stretch and balance exercises *Helps with balance, which worsens with age, posture, and to manage stress.*	*T'ai chi, yoga, and Pilates.*

Managing sleep

As we age, women are more likely than men to experience sleep problems, which become more common and worsen in midlife. Sleep issues affect just under half of all women in the perimenopause, and up to 60 per cent of women post-menopause.

How the menopause impacts sleep

As we age we need less sleep and, typically, we tire and wake up earlier. Menopausal symptoms and changes can also mean that we wake more often and struggle to get back to sleep.

Hormonal changes

Progesterone is mildly sedative. As levels dwindle you may find it harder to fall asleep and to stay asleep. Melatonin, another key sleep hormone, also decreases. Its secretion is influenced by oestrogen and progesterone, so decreasing levels of these compound the problem.

Menopausal symptoms

Heightened anxiety makes it hard to get to sleep and wakes us early. Hot flushes and a need to go to the toilet can interrupt sleep.

Sleep apnoea, snoring, and restless leg syndrome

Hot flushes may increase the risk of sleep apnoea – breathing disturbances in sleep. Weight gain may also play a role as may falling progesterone levels – progesterone affects muscle activity in the throat. Sleep apnoea can cause snoring and gasping and may lead to headaches, insomnia, and anxiety. Restless legs, a tingling sensation in the legs during rest, also increases with age.

Putting in place a healthy sleep regime

Adopting a regular routine, going to bed at the same time each night, will help your body feel ready for sleep. Implementing some of the sleep hygiene measures below will also help to promote restful sleep.

- **Keep your bedroom cool**, well ventilated, quiet, and dark, without light from alarm clocks and phones.
- **Ideally, replace your mattress** every 10 years and invest in comfortable pillows.
- **Wear lightweight, loose clothing** to stay cool at night, or sleep naked. Opt for natural clothing and bedding fibres.
- **Avoid food and drink** for 2–3 hours before bedtime.
- **Avoid coffee** after midday, alcohol in the evening whenever possible, and stimulants, including high-sugar and spicy meals.
- **Try soothing herbal teas** such as chamomile, lemon balm, valerian, and passionflower. Warm milk also contains tryptophan (see below).
- **Opt for low GI foods** (see p.33) and foods high in the amino acid tryptophan – a precursor to the sleep-promoting chemicals melatonin and serotonin – such as turkey, chicken, salmon, tofu, sunflower seeds, chickpeas, buckwheat, dairy, and eggs.
- **Several supplements** aid sleep, including the herbal remedy valerian root; montmorency cherry; magnesium, to calm nerves; and L-theanine.

Managing stress

There is no doubt that the changes that occur to our hormones and bodies during the menopause can make this a stressful transition for many women. Good nutrition, keeping active, and managing sleep are all key to dealing with stress. Finding other outlets, such as talking therapies and relaxation techniques, can also help, and diet and exercise can be tailored to promote relaxation.

How stress affects us

When we experience stress, our adrenal glands produce the stress hormones cortisol and adrenaline – which raise the heart rate and blood sugars to help the body cope in the moment – instead of oestrogen and progesterone, the hormones we need for our health and emotional wellbeing. However, if stress becomes chronic, this can impact our health. In times of stress – whether from a high-sugar diet, feeling overwhelmed, or, in the menopause, from coping with a range of challenging symptoms – our adrenal glands produce high levels of cortisol. This can lead to adrenal fatigue, or "burn out", in turn resulting in reduced energy, fatigue, brain fog, and mood swings.

Stress can also exacerbate existing menopause complaints, such as increased blood pressure and heart rate, headaches, gastric reflux, depression, and anxiety, and, over the long term, an increased risk of heart disease. Stress also affects our immune system, making us more susceptible to illness, infection, and disease. Lastly, but importantly, aside from our physical health, stress affects our relationships, work performance, general wellbeing, and our quality of life.

Looking after your mental health

The damaging effects of stress mean that managing stress in midlife, and in turn preserving your mental health, is one of the key ways to deal with potential menopause symptoms. The following can help.

- **Tailor your diet**. Certain foods help the body to deal with stress. Include oily fish, matcha powder, sweet potatoes, organ meats, eggs, shellfish, and garlic in your diet. Choose herbal teas over stimulants such as coffee and alcohol as caffeine elevates cortisol levels and alcohol interferes with sleep quality.
- **Talk through your concerns**. When possible, share worries with a family member or friend to help you feel supported. It may also be helpful to talk to a healthcare professional or trained counsellor, who will listen and help you work out solutions.
- **Practise relaxation techniques**. Deep breathing exercises, positive thinking, hypnosis, and meditation can all help.
- **Find time for yourself**, whether pursuing a hobby, reading, or having a warm soak in the bath.
- **Prioritize sleep** (see pp.58–59). Restful sleep both reduces stress and helps us cope better with existing stress.
- **Stay active** (see pp.56–57). Make time for exercise and activities. Allow time for your body to recover after exercise, too, as otherwise this can add stress to the body.
- **Consider supplements** if you feel chronic stress is depleting your nutrient store. Magnesium glycinate, omega-3, L-theanine, or herbal remedies such as ashwagandha and rhodiola are some supplements that may help deal with stress.

HRT and other medication

Sometimes, natural solutions for menopause symptoms may not be sufficient or sustainable. In this case, medical solutions such as hormone replacement therapy (HRT) or menopause specific medication for women who cannot take hormones can be useful.

How does HRT help?

HRT administers the hormones oestrogen, progesterone, and sometimes testosterone, either singly or combined, to help relieve symptoms such as hot flushes, night sweats, mood swings, and vaginal dryness. It can also help to prevent osteoporosis post-menopause, and reduces the risk of cardiovascular disease and cognitive decline.

HRT should not be seen as a solution in itself. Looking after your diet and lifestyle should always be your priority, and doing this alongside taking HRT will ensure the best results.

The type of HRT you use will ultimately be a personal choice, taken in consultation with your healthcare provider, who will discuss your symptoms, your current health, any contraindications, and advise you on your choice and the risks. Oestrogen-only HRT is used for women who have had a hysterectomy, where progesterone is not needed to regulate the womb lining. Combined oestrogen and progesterone is for women who have a uterus. Testosterone may also be prescribed alongside these to help with specific symptoms (see opposite).

It can take a few weeks before you feel the initial benefits of HRT and up to three months to feel its full effects. When treatment starts, you may experience side effects such as breast tenderness, nausea, leg cramps, headaches, indigestion, abdominal pain, and vaginal bleeding. These side effects usually disappear within 6–8 weeks. If they persist, you can discuss a change in the type or dose of HRT with your healthcare practitioner.

Oestrogen skin patch
Easy to use, these are usually applied to the abdomen.

Oestrogen gel
Applied to the skin, the dose can be tailored to the individual and their symptoms.

Oestrogen spray
This is quick and easy to use and the dose can be adapted as needed.

Progestogen tablet
This latest form of progesterone has few side effects and is helpful for improving sleep.

Oestrogen implant
A high dose of HRT, this is used when other methods have had less success.

Local vaginal oestrogen
This low-dose HRT is used locally for symptoms such as vaginal dryness.

Oral oestrogen tablet
One of the first forms of HRT, this does carry a higher risk of blood clots.

Progestogen coil
This synthetic progesterone is useful for controlling heavy bleeding.

Testosterone
This is helpful if fatigue, low mood, and lack of libido are persistent problems.

● *Oestrogen*
● *Progesterone*
● *Testosterone*

Types of HRT
HRT delivers steroid hormones (oestrogen, progesterone, and/or testosterone) either orally, via the skin, via an intrauterine device (IUD), or via a subcutaneous implant.

Other medication

When HRT is unsuitable, other types of medication may be suggested.

- **Tibolone** mimics the action of oestrogen and is used to relieve symptoms such as hot flushes, low mood, and reduced sex drive.
- **Antidepressants**, although not licensed for this use, may help with menopausal hot flushes.
- **Clonidine** is a medication that may help to reduce hot flushes and night sweats without affecting your hormone levels.

Natural therapies and other practices

Complementary and natural therapies, such as acupuncture, aromatherapy, and herbal remedies, and techniques such as hypnosis and cognitive behavioural therapy (CBT), can be helpful in the menopause. These can all work alongside diet, lifestyle, and medical solutions such as hormone replacement therapy (HRT, see p.62).

Acupuncture

This form of traditional Chinese medicine, which involves inserting thin needles at acupoints along meridian lines in the body, has been shown to help with a variety of menopausal symptoms. Acupuncture is thought to have a regulating effect on some hormones, which in turn may help reduce the frequency and severity of vasomotor symptoms such as hot flushes. Acupuncture is well documented as a form of pain relief, easing problems such as joint pain. It also works as a relaxation aid, helping to promote restful sleep; and is used to help ease depression and anxiety.

Aromatherapy

Aromatic essential oils are derived from plants and have traditionally been used to improve health and wellbeing. Their relaxing properties can help to ease anxiety in the menopause.

Oils such as fennel, clary sage, and coriander have molecules with an oestrogen-like effect that can help in the menopause, and cooling oils such as peppermint may soothe hot flushes. You can diffuse oils, apply them to pulse points to inhale, or use them in massage, combining the benefits of massage touch therapy with therapeutic oils. Consult a practitioner on which oils to use, how to blend oils for a synergistic effect, and how to use them safely.

Herbal remedies

These use the flowers, fruits, roots, seeds, and stems of plants in herbal preparations to support health and wellbeing. Several herbs may be beneficial in the menopause. Fenugreek seed may help to soothe hot flushes, help balance moods, and ease insomnia. Relaxing herbs such as chamomile, lemon balm, and passionflower can ease anxiety, and St John's wort can help to lift depression. Always consult a qualified herbal practitioner before using herbal remedies, to prepare remedies for you or advise you on how to prepare them, and to direct you on safe use. They can also advise you on contraindications. For example, some herbal remedies, such as St John's wort, can interact with medication. All herbal treatments should be stopped at least two weeks before planned surgery.

Hypnosis

This mind–body therapy works by inducing a deep state of relaxation, from which a therapist can suggest changes to thoughts and behaviours that can be helpful. Studies have shown that hypnotherapy can help to reduce the severity of hot flushes. It can also help women to deal with anxiety in the menopause and improve sleep quality, in turn relieving menopause-related fatigue.

Cognitive behavioural therapy (CBT)

CBT, a form of talking therapy, helps to identify unhelpful thought patterns and feelings that can affect behaviour or, for example, how we feel about certain symptoms. In the menopause, CBT can be used to help with symptoms such as hot flushes, anxiety, and depression. The aim is to help women recognize how their emotional response towards a symptom may intensify the experience of the symptom. Likewise, it can help women to identify triggers for symptoms such as anxiety, so that they can work on and change their reaction to these triggers and work out more positive responses to certain situations.

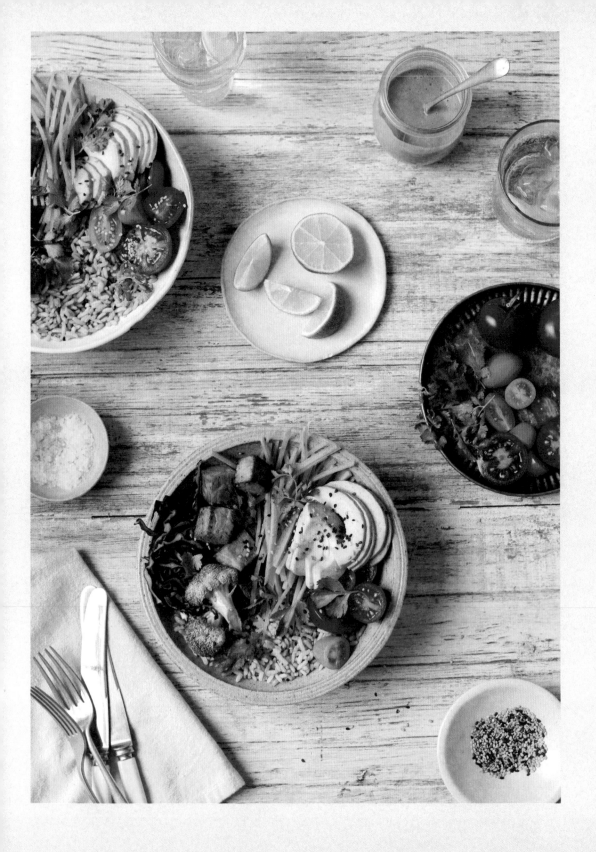

Recipes

for the menopause

An approach to eating

The recipes in this section are split into breakfasts, mains, light bites, desserts and bakes, and drinks. Each meal has a source of protein and fats, with added carbohydrates. Eating similar-sized meals throughout the day, rather than starting with a small breakfast and building up to a large evening meal, steadies blood sugars, supports digestion, and is an ideal way to manage your weight in the menopause.

Breakfasts

This first meal of the day breaks your fast after a night's sleep and sets you up for the morning. However, not everyone feels hungry on waking and some struggle to digest food eaten first thing, so, unless you have a medical condition that means you need to eat breakfast, it is fine to miss this meal if you wish. Your body does need hydrating as soon as you get up, though, so a glass of water first thing is key. If you eat breakfast, the very best start to the day is a savoury meal with at least 20g (³/₄oz) of protein. This will steady blood sugar levels for the rest of the morning and make it unlikely that you will need a snack before lunch. Both savoury and sweet breakfasts are included to help you transition to savoury ones gradually if you wish to do so.

Mains

The recipes in this section are for both lunch and dinner – and for breakfast if you wish. These essential meals need to be substantial to nourish and replenish nutrients. Most of the recipes are designed to add more protein to your diet (see pp.24–27) and include healthy fats. They should help you to stay satiated for longer, so, ideally, you will need to eat only every 4–5 hours, without having energy dips or cravings.

Light bites

Occasionally, you need nourishment outside of meal times, for example, if you prefer to miss breakfast. The light bites here are healthy, low in sugar, and easy to carry if needed, allowing you to eat intuitively when you feel the need without causing sugar levels to yo-yo. Some of the savoury recipes also make great starters or sides.

Desserts and bakes

When blood sugar levels are under control, you can be less inclined to eat dessert. However, you may wish to enjoy desserts and bakes at some family meals, gatherings, and celebrations. The low-sugar, often fruit-based recipes here provide delicious and healthy sweet treats.

Drinks

A small selection of drinks is included, intended as healthy swaps for coffee and tea. Drinks such as breakfast smoothies are not included. Most of us do not feel satiated by drinking foods in liquid form, even if we add the appropriate amount of protein powder, so it is best to avoid replacing a meal with a smoothie or other drink.

A few specifics

Throughout, fan oven temperatures are used. For non-fan ovens, add 20° to celsius temperatures. Unless otherwise stated, milk is either whole dairy, or an unsweetened plant milk, which may affect baking times slightly. Flours are mainly gluten-free (see p.42). On occasion, a specific flour is used, but this can be any gluten-free flour of choice.

Breakfasts

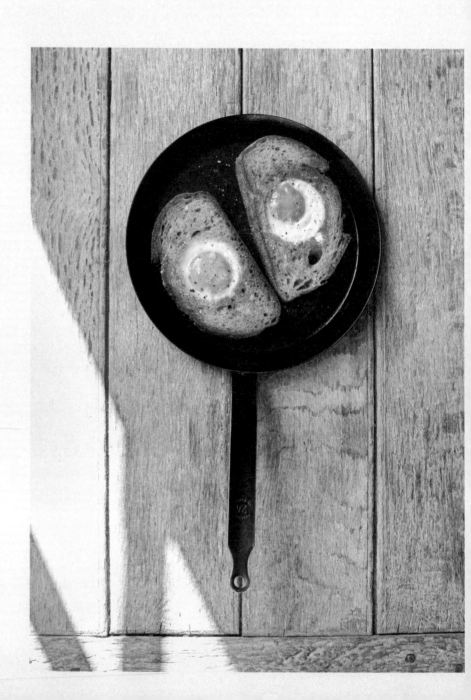

All too often, breakfast is a hurried meal, with little variety from day to day, which, as a result, offers a limited pool of nutrients. The following chapter invites you to take a new approach to this first meal of the day and to treat breakfast as an opportunity to try a range of recipes that will set you up for the morning.

Quick to prep, or easy to make in advance, low-sugar recipes offer delicious sweet and savoury breakfast ideas, with options to enjoy at home or take with you for breakfast on the go. Breakfast favourites, such as porridge and eggs, are given a flavoursome twist with fruits, seeds, and savoury vegetables, and a whole range of inspiring recipes encourages you to take a more adventurous approach to this often-neglected meal. Options to flex recipes are also provided, showing you how to add additional nutrients or adapt a breakfast for a vegetarian or vegan diet. Each recipe provides a sustaining, yet light, complete meal and includes energizing and nutritious ingredients that will leave you feeling satisfied, revitalized, and focused throughout the morning.

Egg muffins

balances hormones • keeps energy levels steady • boosts immunity

These nutrient-dense muffins provide a range of protective antioxidants, while the cholesterol in eggs supports the production of steroid hormones such as oestrogen.

Serves 4
Prep 10 mins
Cook 20 mins

Filling options per person
30g (1oz) cooked mushrooms, 25g (scant 1oz) deseeded and diced red pepper, grated Cheddar
25g (scant 1oz) cooked broccoli, 10g (^{1}/₄oz) goat's cheese, crumbled

25g (scant 1oz) grated courgette, 10g (^{1}/₄oz) goat's cheese, crumbled
30g (1oz) cooked sausage, 25g (scant 1oz) cauliflower rice
10g (^{1}/₄oz) spinach, 10g (^{1}/₄oz) smoked salmon

8–12 eggs (1 egg per muffin)
sea salt and freshly ground black pepper

Preheat the oven to 190°C (400°F/Gas 6). In a silicon muffin tray, add the fillings in the order given above, then add one beaten egg per muffin hole. Season to taste. If you wish, you can prepare the fillings in the muffin tray the night before and store them in the fridge. When ready to cook, simply add the egg and place in the oven.

Depending on the filling, cook for 18–20 minutes, or until the eggs are set. One serving is 2–3 muffins. Enjoy warm or cold.

Flex it – *For extra protein, add Cheddar, feta, or goat's cheese for the options without cheese, or add tofu to any of the veggie fillings.*

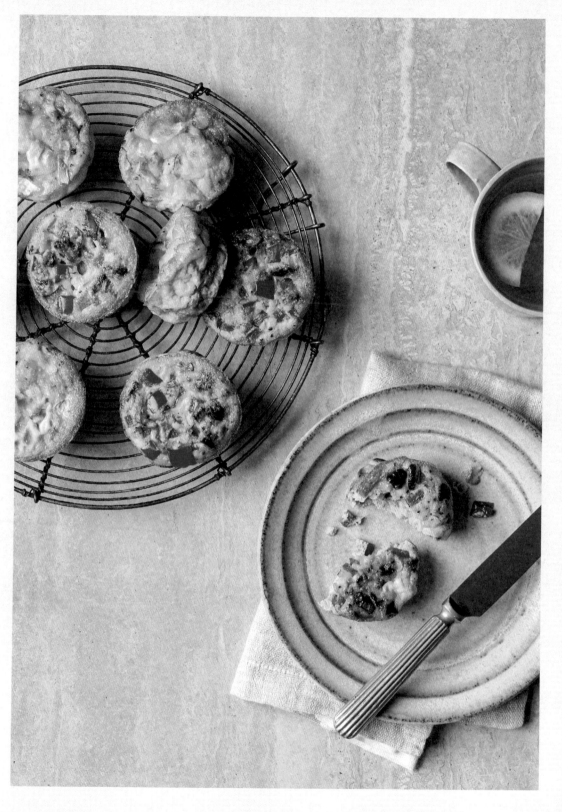

Egg muffins

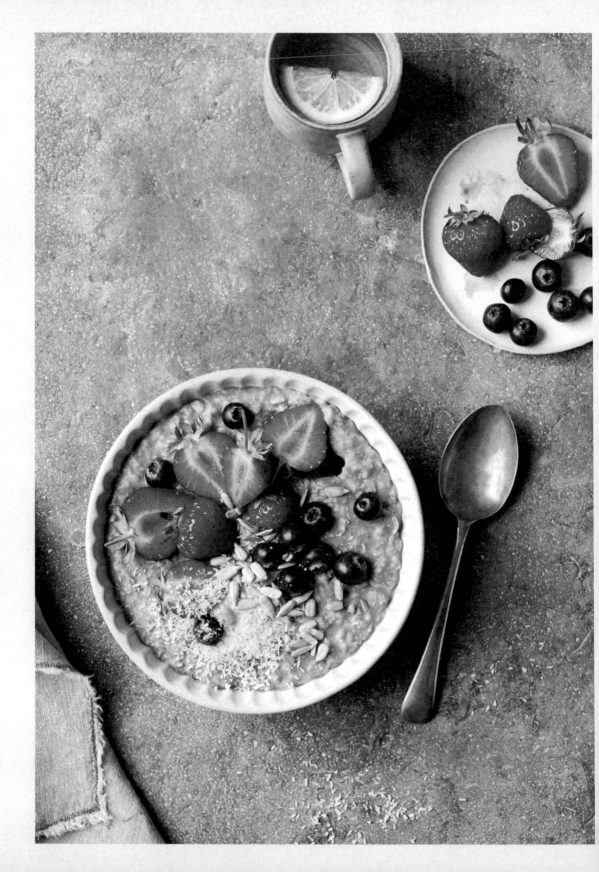

Matcha porridge

energizes • balances moods • calms

Brimming with protective antioxidants, matcha is the perfect morning pick-me-up, releasing its caffeine slowly to provide sustained, calm energy to help combat feelings of fatigue.

Serves 4
Prep 5 mins
Cook 5–7 mins

700ml (1¼ pints) unsweetened
  milk of your choice
1 tbsp matcha green tea powder
200g (7oz) jumbo oats

pinch of sea salt
80g (3oz) blueberries
80g (3oz) strawberries
1 tbsp sunflower seeds
1 tsp desiccated coconut
honey or maple syrup,
  to sweeten (optional)

In a small pan, heat 200ml (7fl oz) of the milk. Transfer the warm milk to a small bowl, add the green tea powder, and whisk well. Set aside.

Add the oats, 450ml (15fl oz) water, and salt to the pan and heat on a medium heat. Once the water has been absorbed, add the remaining milk. Bring to the boil, simmer for 2–3 minutes, then add the green tea milk to the pan and continue to simmer for 1–2 minutes, or until the desired consistency.

Divide the oats equally into four bowls and top up with the berries, sunflower seeds, and coconut. Add a little honey or maple syrup to sweeten, if desired.

Sausage breakfast biscuits

Makes 8
Prep 15 mins
Cook 20 mins

2 tbsp olive oil
**2 pork sausages, about
70g (2¹/₂oz) each, case
removed and meat
roughly chopped**
**½ red pepper, deseeded
and diced**
**1 garlic clove, finely
chopped**
80g (3oz) almond flour
1 tsp baking powder
10 sage leaves
2 eggs
80g (3oz) Cheddar, grated

**helps manage weight • promotes muscle health
• helps calm hot flushes**

These high-protein breakfast bites promote
muscle health and keep hunger at bay, reducing
the urge to snack. The addition of sage may have
a calming effect on hot flushes.

Preheat the oven to 190°C (400°F/Gas 6) and line
a baking sheet with parchment paper.

Heat a frying pan over a medium heat, then add the
olive oil, sausages, pepper, and garlic. Stir well until
the sausage is cooked through and the peppers are
softened, for about 10 minutes. Set aside.

In a medium bowl, combine the flour, baking powder,
and sage. Add the eggs, half the cheese, and the
sausage mix and combine well.

Make balls, using about 45g (1¹/₂oz) of the mixture for
each one. Place the balls on the parchment paper and
press down gently on each one to flatten it. Sprinkle
the remaining cheese over the balls.

Bake for 9–10 minutes, or until the biscuits are cooked
through and slightly brown on the bottom. Serve warm.

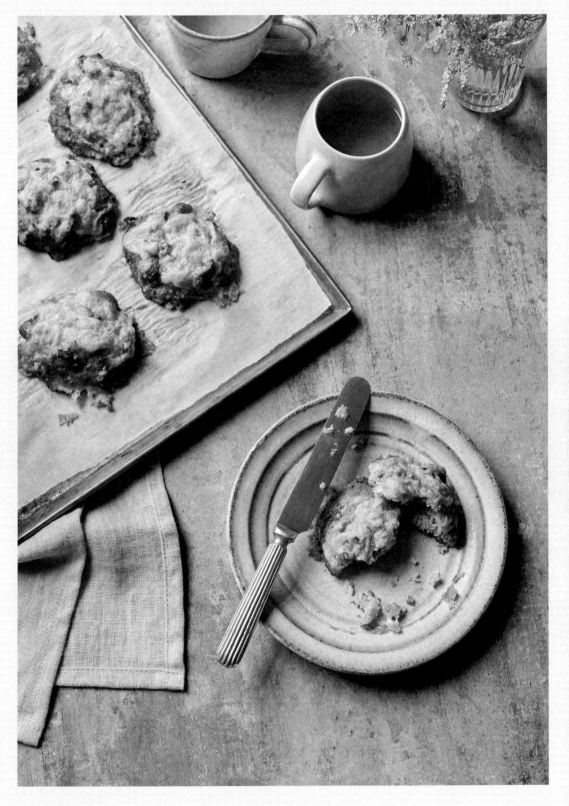

Sausage breakfast biscuits

Strawberry *and* tahini overnight oats

Serves 4
Prep 5 mins
Rest 6 hours

200g (7oz) jumbo oats
700ml (1¼ pints) unsweetened
  milk of your choice
80g (3oz) chia seeds
120g (4½oz) tahini
zest of 1 lemon
1 tbsp balsamic vinegar
300g (10oz) strawberries,
  chopped
cinnamon or drizzle of honey,
  to sweeten (optional)

supports digestion • balances mood • keeps energy levels steady

This refreshing breakfast includes tahini, a good source of calcium for strong bones, and is also high in fibre and healthy fats to satisfy the appetite.

Place the oats, milk, chia seeds, tahini, lemon zest, and balsamic vinegar in a kilner jar and mix well. Cover and place in the fridge overnight, or for at least 6 hours.

Divide the oats between four bowls and top with the strawberries. Add cinnamon and/or a drizzle of honey to sweeten, if desired.

Smoked salmon *and* egg *on* avocado toast

Serves 4
Prep 15 mins

2 avocados
juice of 1 lemon
sea salt and freshly
    ground black pepper
4 large slices of bread,
    ideally gluten-free,
    toasted
2 tbsp butter or ghee
8 eggs, beaten
4 slices of smoked salmon
1 tbsp finely chopped
    chives
tomatoes or cucumber,
    diced, to serve

Flex it – *For a vegetarian option that keeps some of the omega-3 benefits, substitute the salmon with wilted spinach and flaxseeds.*

provides sustained energy • supports cognition • aids memory

As well as providing protein, eggs are high in choline, which, together with omega-3s in salmon and healthy fats in avocado, promotes healthy brain function in the menopause years.

Put the avocados and lemon juice in a bowl, season, and mash together with a fork.

Place the toast on serving plates then use the fork to spread the mashed avocado over each slice.

Melt the butter or ghee in a large, heavy-based frying pan over a medium heat. Add the eggs and cook for about 4 minutes, gently stirring occasionally, until just set. Spoon the eggs evenly over the avocado.

Place the salmon on top of the egg and scatter over the chives. Serve with diced tomatoes or diced cucumber on the side.

(photographed overleaf)

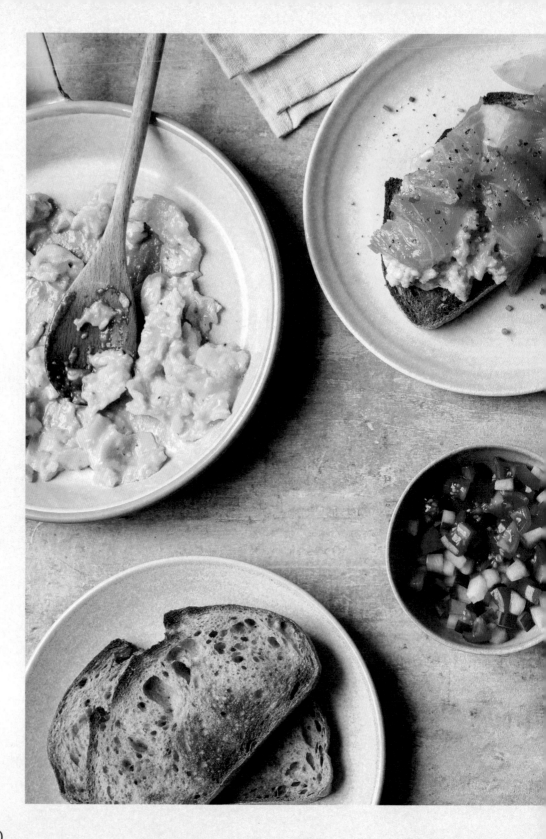

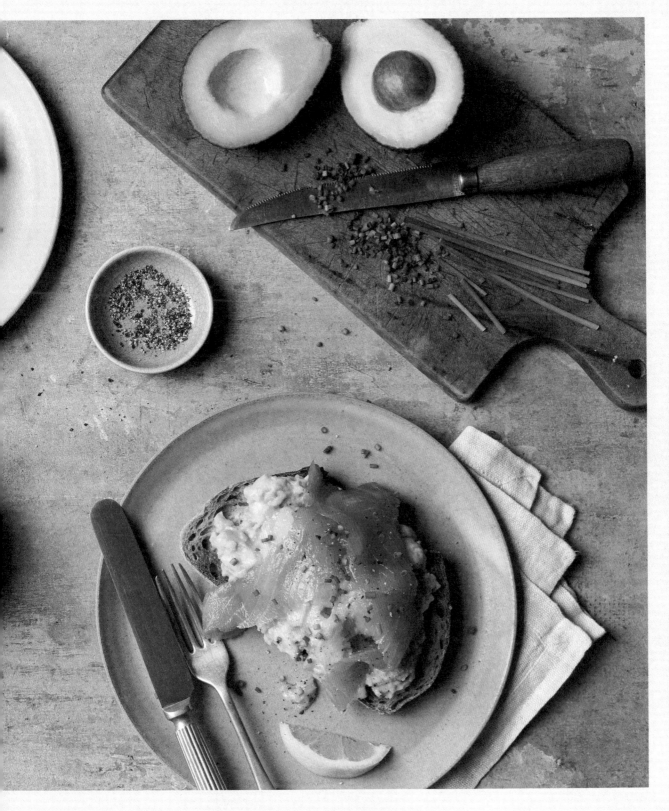

Smoked salmon and egg on avocado toast

Orange *and* turmeric overnight oats

Serves 4
Prep 5–10 mins
Rest 6 hours

200g (7oz) jumbo oats
2 tbsp chia seeds
475ml (15½ fl oz)
  unsweetened milk
  of your choice
2 tsp turmeric
1 tsp cinnamon
pinch of sea salt
1–2 navel oranges, zest,
  juice of ½ an orange,
  and segments
4 tbsp pumpkin seeds
4 tbsp pomegranate seeds
honey or maple syrup, to
  sweeten (optional)

balances moods • helps manage weight • promotes healthy joints

This cooling oat dish keeps you full and helps regulate blood sugars, in turn managing weight and fluctuating moods; while turmeric adds anti-inflammatory properties to soothe joint pain.

Place the oats, chia seeds, milk, spices, salt, orange juice, and half the orange zest in a kilner jar. Stir well to combine. Seal and place in the fridge overnight, or for at least 6 hours.

Chop the remaining orange into segments. Divide the overnight oats into bowls and add the orange segments, the remaining zest, and the pumpkin and pomegranate seeds. Add a little honey or maple syrup to sweeten, if desired.

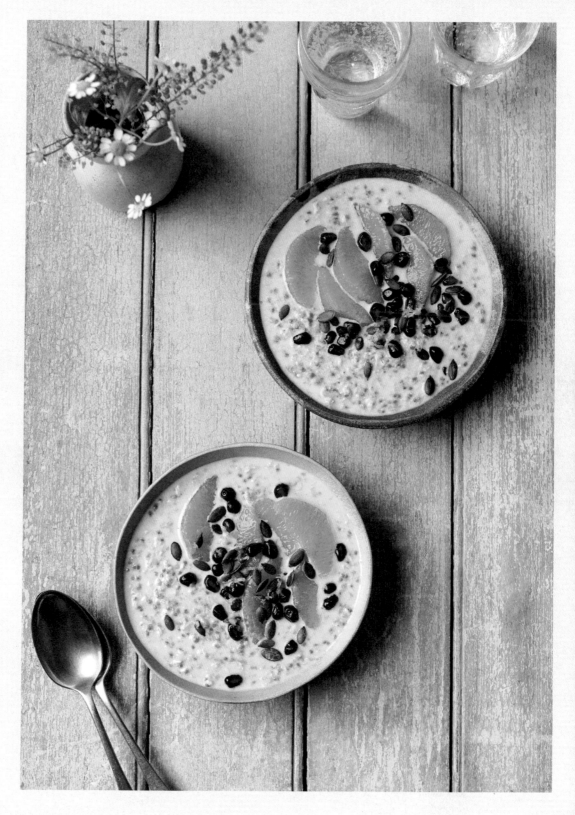

Orange and turmeric overnight oats

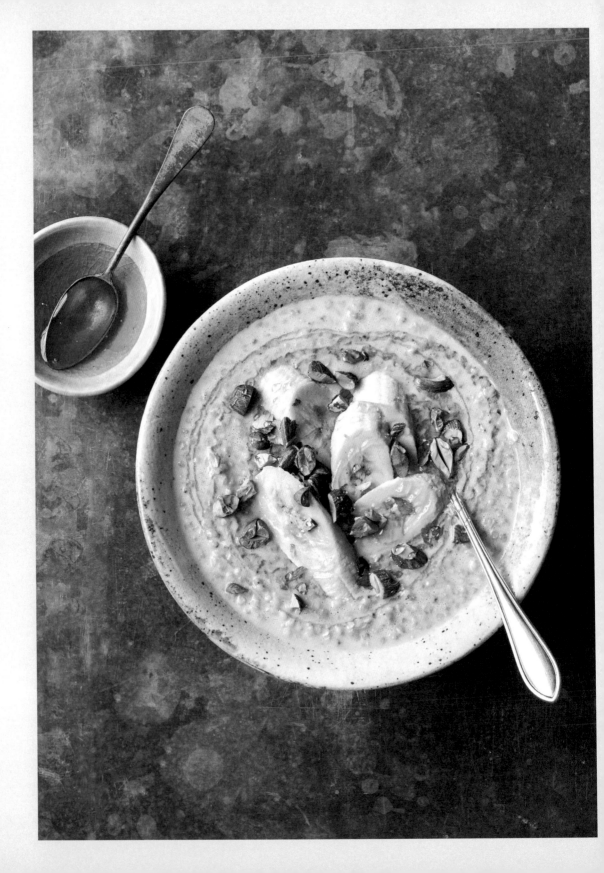

Banana buckwheat porridge

provides sustained energy • eases anxiety • calms

Buckwheat and bananas contain many B vitamins, important for managing stress and maintaining energy levels in the menopause, while crunchy almonds supply magnesium, levels of which are often low in midlife.

Serves 4
Prep 5 mins
Cook 15 mins

200g (7oz) buckwheat groats
1¹/₂ tbsp cinnamon

1¹/₂ tbsp clear honey
240ml (8fl oz) unsweetened milk of your choice
2 bananas
40g (1¹/₂oz) almonds, chopped

Place the buckwheat and 500ml (16fl oz) water in a small pan over a medium heat. Bring to the boil, then cover and simmer for 10–15 minutes, or until the water is absorbed and the buckwheat is cooked.

Add the cinnamon, honey, and milk and stir until well combined.

Divide between four bowls, slice half a banana over each bowl, then sprinkle over the almonds to serve.

Cinnamon *and* seeds breakfast bowl

Serves 4
Prep 10 mins
Cook 5 mins

500ml (16fl oz)
   unsweetened almond
   milk, or unsweetened
   milk of your choice
240g (8¹/₂oz) chia seeds
40g (1¹/₂oz) unsweetened
   shredded coconut, plus
   extra for serving
60g (2oz) ground flaxseeds
1 tbsp cinnamon
80g (3oz) mixed nuts,
   chopped

Flex it – *Top with fruit for extra sweetness, antioxidants, and fibre.*

supports digestion • helps calm hot flushes • keeps energy levels steady

This easy-to-digest, grain-free porridge is high in phytoestrogens from the flaxseeds, to ease hot flushes, while cinnamon helps to keep blood sugar levels on an even keel, avoiding energy dips.

Heat the milk in a small pan over a medium heat, until hot but not boiling. Take off the heat, then add the chia seeds, coconut, flaxseeds, and cinnamon. Stir well until the porridge has thickened.

Leave the porridge to sit for 1–2 minutes to allow the chia seeds and flaxseeds to absorb more milk. Transfer the porridge to bowls and serve topped with the nuts and extra coconut.

Chocolate, courgette, *and* ginger muffins

Makes 4
Prep 15 mins
Cook 18–20 mins
Rest 15 mins

70g (2¹/₂oz) ground almonds
1¹/₂ tbsp 100 per cent cocoa
   powder
¹/₄ tsp sea salt
¹/₄ tsp bicarbonate of soda
1¹/₂ tbsp olive oil
2 tbsp maple syrup
1 egg
1 small courgette, about
   130g (4³/₄oz), grated
2cm (³/₄in) piece of ginger,
   finely grated

supports digestion • promotes healthy joints • helps hydrate

Refreshing courgettes make these moreish breakfast muffins a hydrating treat. Olive oil adds moistness and supports joint health, while the addition of ginger helps quell any nausea.

Preheat the oven to 180°C (400°F/Gas 6). Place all the ingredients, except the courgette and ginger, in a large bowl and mix together. Add the courgette and ginger and combine well.

Spoon the muffin batter into 4 silicon muffin tray compartments and bake for 18 minutes, or until the centre of the muffin is cooked and an inserted skewer comes out clean. Allow the muffins to cool completely before serving.

Mushroom *and* thyme porridge

Serves 4
Prep 10 mins
Cook 15 mins

2 tbsp olive oil
1 onion, finely sliced
250g (9oz) mushrooms,
thinly sliced
10g (¼oz) sprigs of thyme,
leaves only, plus a few
extra to garnish
200g (7oz) jumbo oats
2 tbsp tamari soy sauce

Flex it – *To top up your protein, add some grated Parmesan or Cheddar, crumble over feta, or add a poached or scrambled egg.*

boosts immunity • helps calm hot flushes • has anti-inflammatory properties

High in immune-supporting beta glucans, mushrooms help protect the body from low-grade inflammation in the menopause. Flavourful tamari contains a key phytoestrogen, to ease hot flushes.

Heat a frying pan over a medium heat. Add the olive oil, allow to warm, then add the onion and cook until soft and translucent, about 5 minutes.

Add the mushrooms and cook until soft. Add the thyme, mixing it with the mushrooms, then set aside.

In a medium pan, add the oats and 950ml (1½ pints) of water. Bring to the boil then simmer for 5 minutes, or until the desired consistency. Add the tamari. Stir well.

Divide the porridge between four bowls or plates and top with the mushrooms.

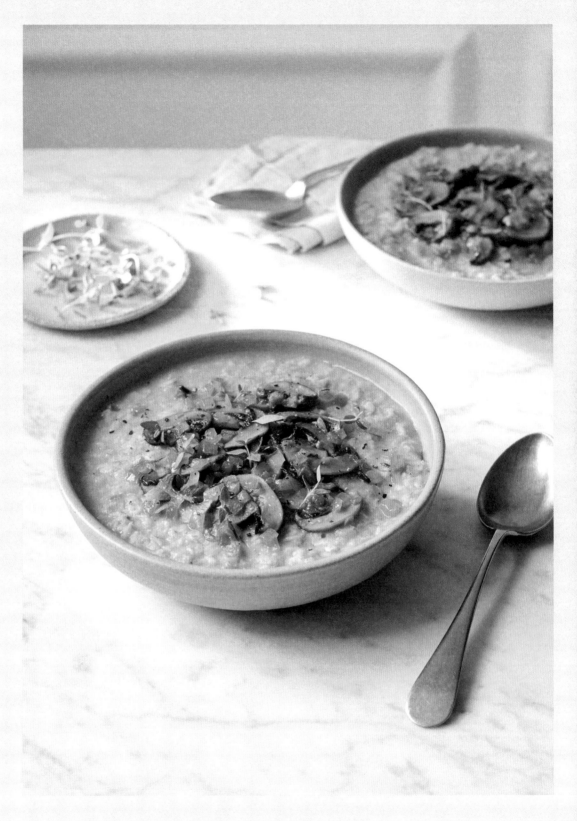

Mushroom and thyme porridge

Granola

**helps manage weight • keeps energy levels steady
• supports heart health**

High in proteins and fats and with minimal sugar, this simple
granola mix provides a nutritionally complete meal to set you up
for the morning. Eating calming oats regularly supports heart
health during the menopause years.

Makes 12 servings
Prep 5 mins
Cook 20–25 mins
Rest 15 mins

200g (7oz) jumbo oats
70g (2$\frac{1}{2}$oz) almonds
70g (2$\frac{1}{2}$oz) pecan nuts
70g (2$\frac{1}{2}$oz) hemp seeds
120ml (4fl oz) coconut oil, melted
60ml (2fl oz) maple syrup
$\frac{1}{2}$ tsp sea salt

Preheat the oven to 190°C (400°F/Gas 6). Line a baking tray with
parchment paper. Place all the ingredients in a large bowl and
combine well.

Pour the mixture onto the baking tray and bake for 20–25 minutes,
stirring a few times to achieve an even colour. Leave to cool
completely. Store in an airtight container at room temperature
for up to 1 month.

Decadent chocolate avocado brownie

balances moods • keeps energy levels steady • supports heart health

This breakfast treat provides sweetness without causing blood sugar levels to spike. High in proteins and heart-healthy fats, this will keep you full and satisfied through to lunch.

Serves 4
Prep 15 mins
Cook 17–20 mins
Rest 15 mins

1 avocado
2 eggs
1 tsp vanilla extract

70g (2^1/$_2$oz) coconut sugar
zest of 1 lime
40g (1^1/$_2$oz) coconut oil, melted
50g (1^3/$_4$oz) almond flour
40g (1^1/$_2$oz) 100 per cent cacao powder
1 tsp bicarbonate of soda
^{1}/$_2$ tsp salt

Preheat the oven to 190°C (400°F/Gas 6). Line a 19 x 14cm (7^1/$_2$ x 5^1/$_2$in) baking tin with parchment paper. Mash the avocado and place the avocado, eggs, vanilla extract, coconut sugar, and lime zest in a large mixing bowl. Whisk the ingredients with a hand-held blender until well combined.

Add the remaining ingredients and mix until well combined. Pour the mixture into the baking tin and bake for 17–20 minutes, or until cooked and an inserted skewer comes out almost clean. Leave the brownies to cool before slicing.

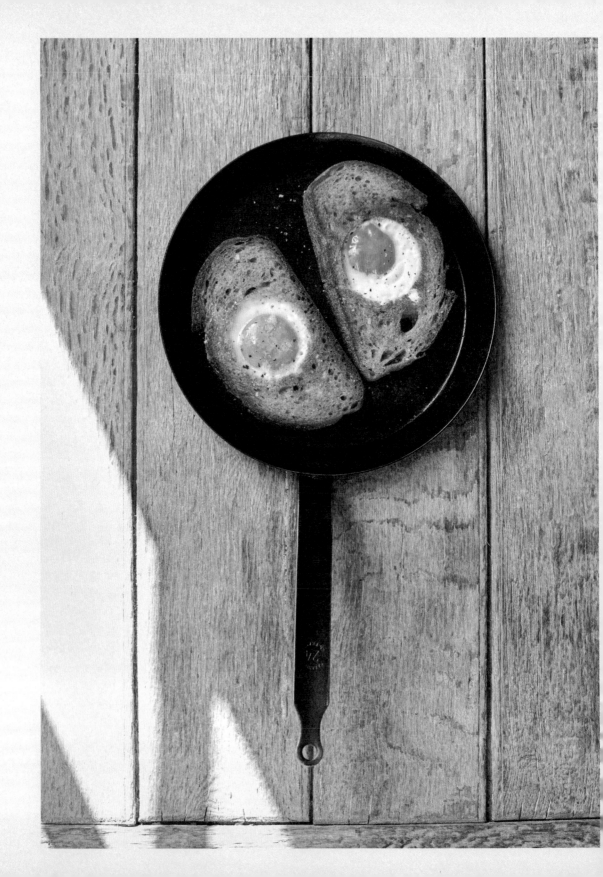

Egg *in a* hole

**keeps energy levels steady • balances moods
• helps manage weight**

This simple eggy breakfast provides protein to keep you going through the morning, helping to avoid fluctuating moods and removing the urge to snack.

Serves 4
Prep 2 mins
Cook 7 mins

**4 large slices of bread, ideally
gluten-free
10g ('/₄oz) butter or ghee
4 eggs
side salad, to serve (optional)**

Heat a frying pan over a medium heat. Cut a large circle or square in the middle of each slice of bread. Melt the butter or ghee in the pan, then add the bread slices. Crack an egg into each hole while pressing down on the borders of the bread to make sure the egg white doesn't run under the bread.

After about 2 minutes, gently turn each slice. For a runny yolk, cook for another 2 minutes, or a little longer for a non-runny yolk. Serve straight away, with a side salad if desired.

Flex it – *For a non-vegetarian option, add two rashers of bacon.*

Za'atar tartine

promotes bone health • supports digestion • promotes muscle health

Refreshing labneh – strained yogurt – is a good source of filling protein, essential for muscle and bone health, and contains probiotics, supporting a healthy gut microbiome.

Serves 4
Prep 5 mins

2 tbsp olive oil
4 tbsp za'atar spice mix
4 large slices of bread, ideally
   gluten-free

140g (5oz) labneh yogurt, shop-bought or prepare by straining unsweetened Greek yogurt through a muslin for 12 hours

Put the olive oil and za'atar in a small bowl and stir to combine. (This mixture can be prepared in advance and refrigerated for up to 1 month.)

Toast the bread then divide the labneh evenly on top of each piece of toast and top each slice with 1 tablespoon of the za'atar mix. Enjoy while the toast is warm.

Flex it – *For a vegan option, swap the labneh in this recipe for a thick unsweetened non-dairy yogurt.*

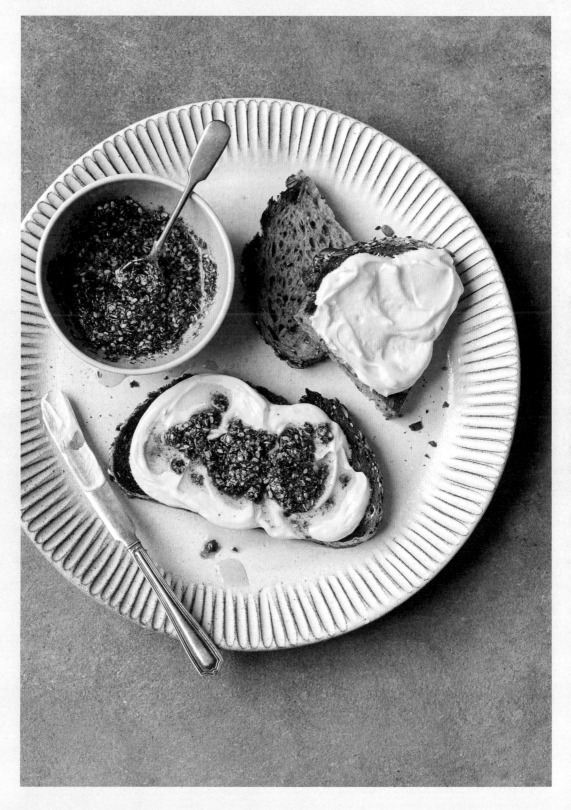

Za'atar tartine

Mains

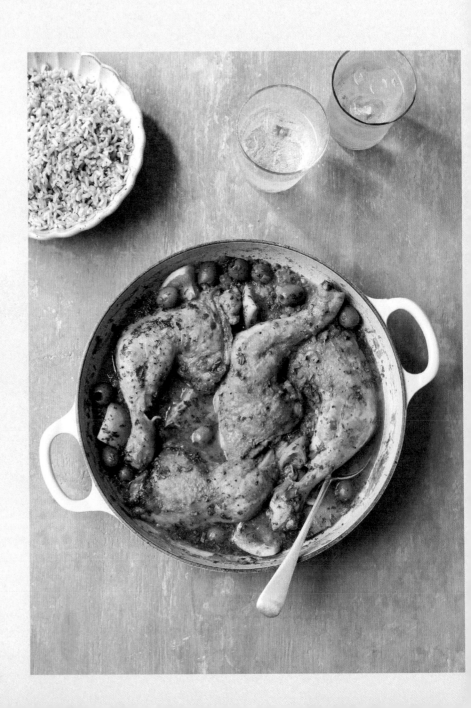

Main meals are often thought of as end-of-the-day fare when we sit down to enjoy our biggest meal of the day. If previous meals have been relatively small, this can fuel hunger and tempt us to indulge in portion sizes that are larger than needed, or to refill plates for seconds. Instead, eating more evenly portioned dishes throughout the day helps to balance blood sugar levels and keeps us satisfied between meals.

This appetizing and versatile selection of main meals provides inspiration for family lunches and suppers throughout the week. Dishes are beautifully simple and easy to rustle up – many taking less than an hour from prep to plate – making them easy options for both lunch and dinner. A handful of slow-cooked dishes also offers ideas for more leisurely weekend meals or celebratory dishes.

The recipes cater for meat, vegetarian, and vegan diets, with flex ideas offering easy ways to remove or add meat and dairy without dropping key nutrients. Recipes range from uncomplicated, but nutritionally dense, dishes such as omelettes and satisfying salads, to traditional classics such as roast chicken and baked cod. There is also a range of delicious and innovative ingredient combos, encouraging you to broaden your repertoire and diversify your nutritional intake.

Scallops *with* sweet potato purée

Serves 4
Prep 10 mins
Cook 35–45 mins

600g (1lb 5oz) sweet
   potatoes, peeled and
   diced
30g (1oz) butter or ghee
$^1/_4$ tsp sea salt, plus extra
   for additional seasoning
150g (5$^1/_2$oz) prosciutto,
   sliced into small pieces
1$^1/_2$ tbsp olive oil
30g (1oz) sage
400g (14oz) scallops,
   or 2–4 per person

supports metabolism • promotes bone health • helps calm hot flushes • eases anxiety

Scallops contain iodine, vital for thyroid and bone health. Starchy sweet potatoes release energy slowly and provide B vitamins to help manage anxiety, and sage can help to soothe hot flushes.

Bring a large pan of water to the boil, add the sweet potato, and cook until tender. Drain and mash into a smooth purée with the butter or ghee and salt.

Heat a large frying pan over a medium heat. Add the prosciutto and cook for a few minutes each side, or until crisp. Remove from the pan and set aside. Using the same pan, add half of the olive oil and the sage. Fry until crispy, then remove and set aside.

Season the scallops with salt. Return the pan to a medium heat and add the remaining olive oil. Add the scallops and cook for 3–4 minutes on each side.

Assemble the plates with the sweet potato purée, then top with the scallops, sage, and prosciutto.

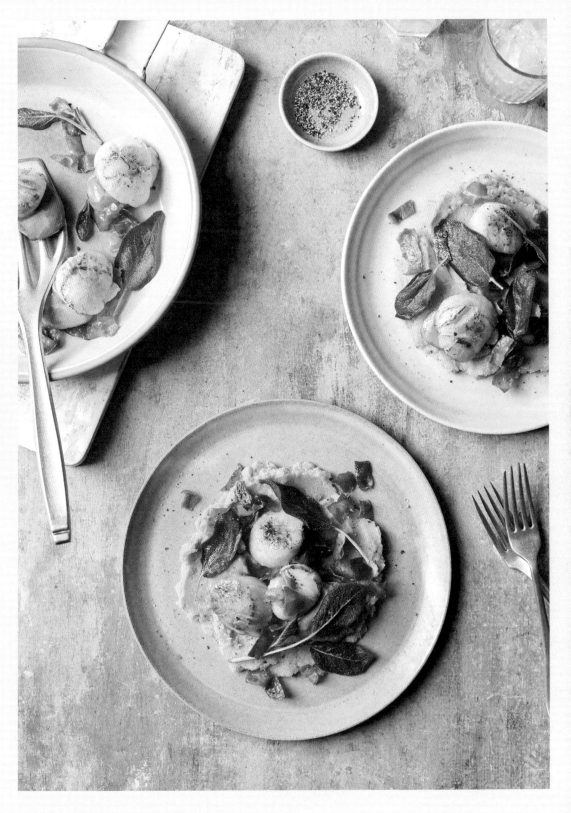

Scallops with sweet potato purée

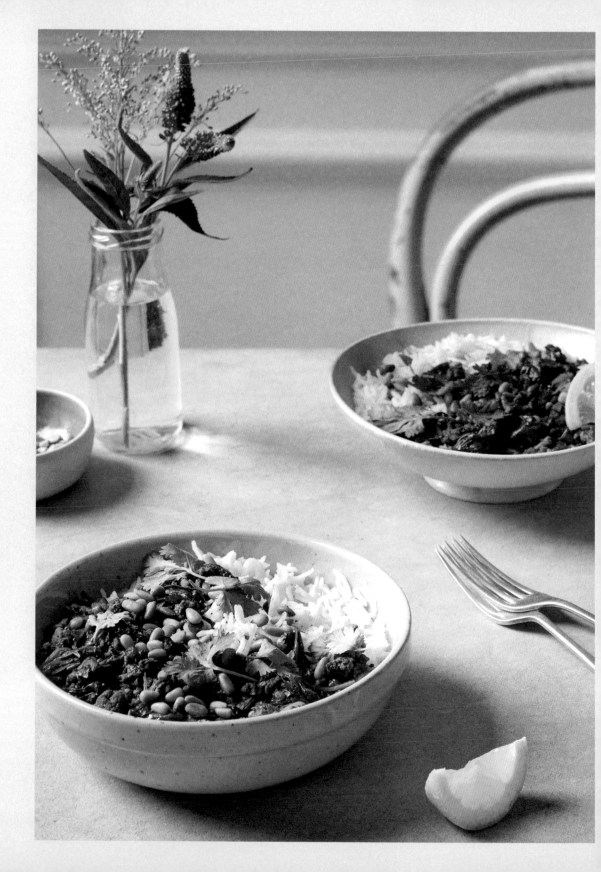

Beef, spinach, *and* spices *with* rice

supports bone and muscle health • provides sustained energy

This beef and spinach combo is a perfectly balanced nutrient-dense dish, high in muscle-building protein, energizing iron, plus vitamins D and K for bone health.

Serves 4
Prep 5 mins
Cook 20–25 mins

200g (7oz) basmati rice
15g (½oz) butter or ghee
1 large onion, finely chopped

500g (1lb 2oz) minced beef
1 tbsp Lebanese 7 spice
1 tbsp allspice
350g (12oz) baby spinach
juice of 1 lemon
25g (scant 1oz) pine nuts, roasted
coriander, to garnish

Cook the rice according to the packet instructions. In the meantime, heat a large frying pan over a medium heat and add the butter or ghee. Once melted, add the onion and fry, stirring, for 5 minutes, or until the onion is translucent.

Turn the heat up to high and add the beef. Using two wooden spoons, stir the beef and separate it into small pieces in the pan. Cook for 5 minutes, or until the meat is browned.

Add the spices and combine with the meat. Turn the heat to low then add half the spinach and combine. Once the spinach is wilted, add the remaining spinach and mix well. Simmer for 8–10 minutes. Turn off the heat and add the lemon juice, stirring to combine.

Divide the rice between the plates, add the beef and spinach, sprinkle over the pine nuts, and garnish with the coriander.

Blushing octopus

Serves 4
Prep 10 mins
Cook 90 mins
Rest 10 mins

sea salt and freshly
  ground black pepper
1 large onion, roughly
  sliced
1 bay leaf
1 large octopus, about
  3.5–5kg (7–10lb), frozen
  then defrosted
100ml (3$\frac{1}{2}$fl oz) olive oil,
  plus extra virgin olive
  oil for drizzling
80g (3oz) capers
2 tbsp paprika
2 tbsp flat-leaf parsley,
  chopped
new potatoes, green
  salad, and tomato salsa,
  to serve

supports heart health • promotes healthy joints • aids cognition

Octopus contains omega-3 fatty acids, key for brain and joint health, while paprika provides vitamin E and iron for healthy blood vessels and the anti-inflammatory compound capsaicin.

Fill a large pan with water, add a pinch of salt, and bring to the boil. Add the onion and bay leaf, then add the octopus and boil for 90 minutes, turning the octopus every 30 minutes.

Remove the octopus from the water and allow it to cool on a tray for 10 minutes. Discard the head and slice the tentacles into 5mm ($\frac{1}{4}$in) rounds.

Heat the olive oil in a large frying pan. In batches, fry the octopus pieces for a few minutes, adding more olive oil if needed.

Arrange the octopus on a serving plate, drizzle with olive oil, and add the capers. Sprinkle with the paprika, season, and scatter over the parsley. Serve straight away with some new potatoes, a green salad, and a tomato salsa.

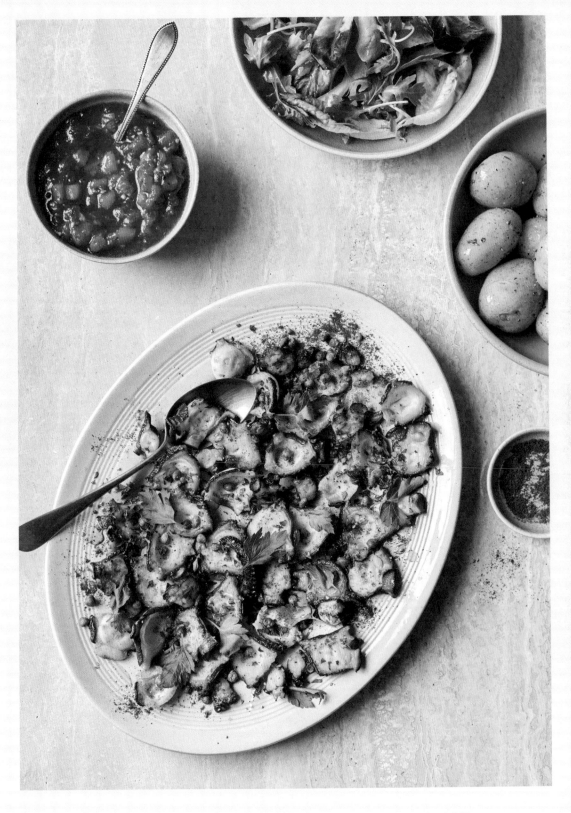

Blushing octopus

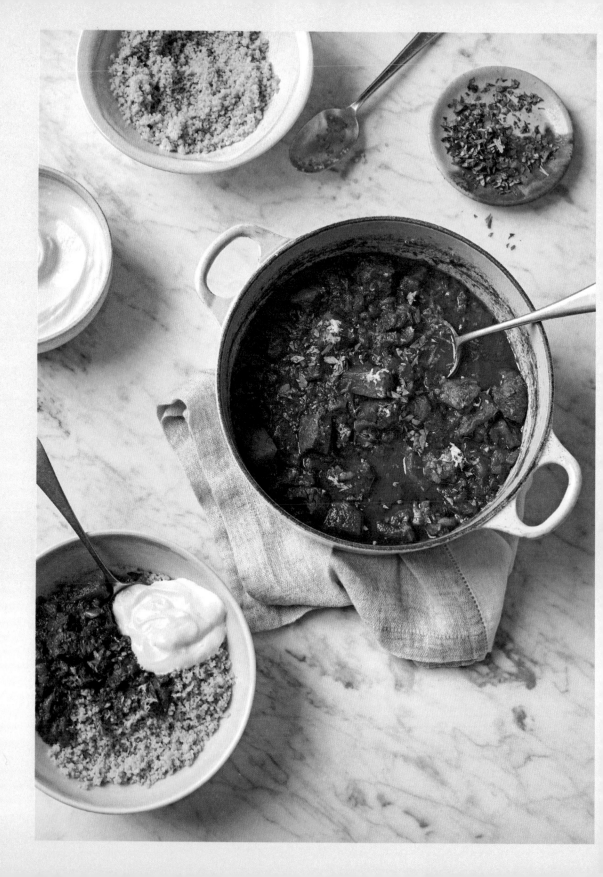

Lamb tagine

Serves 4
Prep 20 mins
Cook 90 mins

2 tbsp olive oil
1 large onion, finely chopped
2 garlic cloves, finely chopped
1 tbsp ras el hanout
1 tsp ground coriander
600g (1lb 5oz) leg of lamb,
    diced into 2cm (³⁄₄in) pieces,
    excess fat trimmed
200g (7oz) butternut squash,
    diced
100g (3¹⁄₂oz) soft dried apricots
400g can chopped tomatoes
500ml (16fl oz) bone broth
    (see p.216)
sea salt and freshly ground
    black pepper
zest of 1 lemon
coriander leaves, chopped,
    to serve
quinoa and yogurt, to serve

Flex it – *For extra protein,
add a can of chickpeas, or for a
vegetarian dish, add 2 cans of
chickpeas and reduce the oven
cooking time accordingly.*

supports muscle health • supports digestion • boosts immunity

Protein-dense lamb helps maintain muscle health, while mineral-rich bone broth has gut-healing properties, in turn strengthening immunity.

Heat the oil in a flameproof casserole dish, add the onion, and cook for 5 minutes, until softened. Add the garlic and spices and cook for another 2 minutes, stirring well.

Add the lamb, squash, and apricots, pour over the tomatoes and bone broth, season well, and bring to the boil. Place the lid on the casserole and cook for about 1 hour on a low heat, stirring occasionally. Remove the lid and cook for a further 30 minutes. Check the seasoning. Sprinkle over the lemon zest and coriander and serve in warm bowls with quinoa and yogurt.

Mussels in white wine

Serves 4
Prep 10 mins
Cook 15 mins

1 tbsp butter or ghee
2 shallots, thinly sliced
2 garlic cloves, thinly sliced
400ml (14fl oz) dry white
  wine
2kg (4$\frac{1}{2}$lb) mussels,
  cleaned
25g (scant 1oz) flat-leaf
  parsley, finely chopped,
  to garnish
potato wedges, to serve

**boosts immunity • supports metabolism
• promotes bone health**

Like all seafood, mussels are rich in iodine, helpful for bone health and key for the metabolism of thyroid hormones. In addition, garlic and shallots have immune-boosting properties.

In a large pot with a lid, melt the butter or ghee over a medium heat. Once the butter begins to foam, stir in the shallots and garlic and cook until softened, about 5 minutes.

Add the wine and the mussels, give them a good stir, and cover the pot with the lid.

After a few minutes, turn and mix the mussels to allow them to open easily. Replace the lid and cook for a few more minutes, until all the mussels are opened, discarding any that remain shut. Sprinkle with the parsley and serve immediately with potato wedges on the side.

Beef bourguignon

Serves 4
Prep 15 mins
Cook 2 hours 30 mins

4 tbsp olive oil
1 onion, finely chopped
2 garlic cloves, crushed
1kg (2¼lb) braising beef, cut
   into 4–5cm (1½–2in) chunks,
   fat or sinew trimmed
4 carrots, roughly chopped
2 tbsp tomato purée
200ml (7fl oz) bone broth
   (see p.216)
2 large bay leaves
3 sprigs of thyme
sea salt and freshly ground
   black pepper
10g (¼oz) butter or ghee
300g (10oz) small chestnut
   mushrooms, halved
2 tbsp cornflour

keeps energy levels steady • boosts immunity • eases anxiety • supports digestion

Beef supplies vitamin B12, often low in the menopause, but key for brain health, energy, and for coping with stress. Mineral-rich bone broth aids metabolism, immunity, and heart and gut health.

Heat a large flameproof casserole dish over a low heat, add 2 tablespoons of the olive oil, and cook the onion until softened, about 5 minutes. Add the garlic and cook for another minute. Add the remaining olive oil and fry the beef until browned.

Add the carrots, tomato purée, bone broth, and the herbs. Season and bring to a simmer. Stir, cover with a lid, and cook for about 1½ hours on a low heat.

In the meantime, heat a large frying pan over a medium heat. Melt the butter or ghee, add the mushrooms, and cook until golden. Set aside. Place the cornflour and 2 tablespoons of water in a bowl and mix until smooth.

Stir in the cornflour mixture, add the mushrooms, and cook for another 45 minutes, or until the beef is tender and the sauce has thickened. Remove the thyme sprigs and serve.

Bacon, mushroom, *and* egg cauliflower bowl

balances hormones • promotes muscle health • energizes

Full of muscle-supporting, sustaining protein, this satisfying dish works well for lunch, dinner, or breakfast. Part of the cruciferous family, cauliflower supports liver function to ensure healthy hormone metabolism.

Serves 4
Prep 15 mins
Cook 20 mins

8 slices of preservative-free bacon
4 tbsp olive oil

1 large onion, thinly sliced
500g (1lb 2oz) mushrooms, finely chopped
2 tbsp tamari soy sauce
20g ($^3/_4$oz) thyme, leaves only
600g (1lb 5oz) cauliflower, grated
8 eggs

Heat a frying pan to a medium heat and cook the bacon as desired – tender to crisp. Set aside.

Add 1 tablespoon of the olive oil and cook the onion for a few minutes. Add another tablespoon of the olive oil then add the mushrooms and tamari and cook until tender. Add the thyme and combine well. Remove and set aside. Add the remaining olive oil and cook the cauliflower for 5–7 minutes, stirring well. Return the mushrooms to the pan and combine with the cauliflower.

Poach, scramble, or fry the eggs as desired. Divide the cauliflower between the serving plates, together with the eggs and bacon.

Flex it – *For a vegetarian option, remove the bacon.*

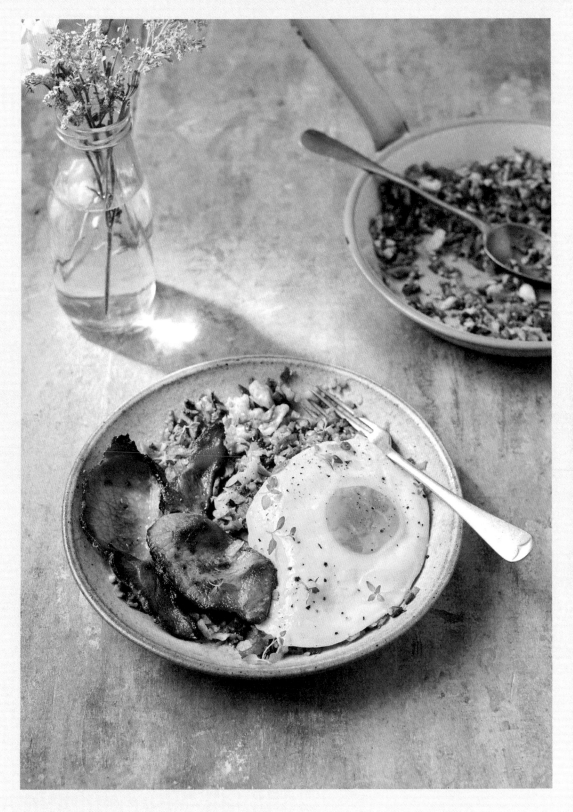

Bacon, mushroom, and egg cauliflower bowl

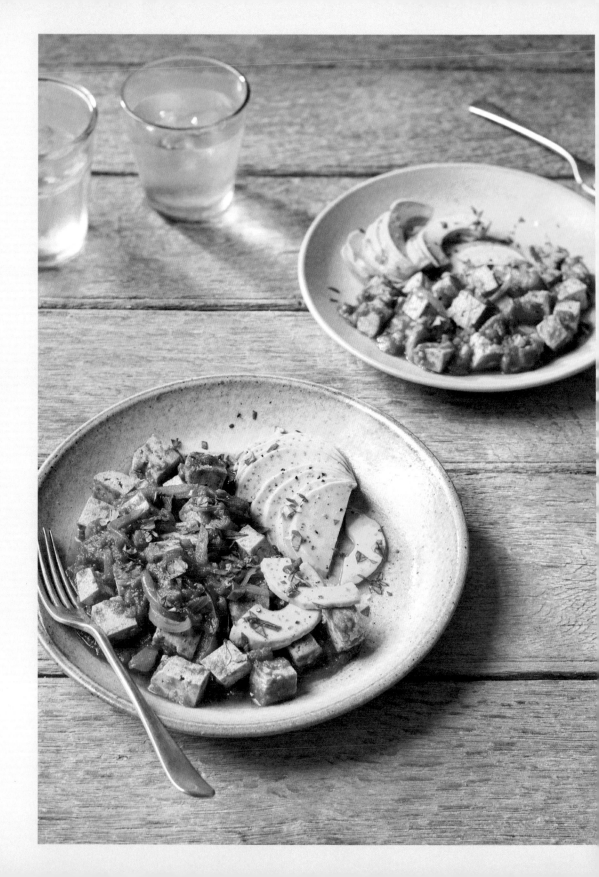

Tofu shakshuka

helps calm hot flushes • provides sustained energy • promotes bone health

High in filling protein, tofu includes phytoestrogens, to relieve hot flushes. In addition, the cooked tomatoes provide lycopene, thought to reduce the risk of osteoporosis post-menopause.

Serves 4
Prep 10 mins
Cook 30 mins

1 tbsp olive oil
1 onion, sliced
2 garlic cloves, crushed
1 red pepper, deseeded and
    thinly sliced
2 tbsp paprika
1 tsp cumin
2 x 400g can chopped tomatoes
sea salt and freshly ground
    black pepper
400g (14oz) firm tofu, pat-dried
    and diced
2 tbsp parsley, finely chopped
1 avocado, pitted and sliced

Preheat the oven to 190°C (400°F/Gas 6). Heat the olive oil in a flameproof casserole over a medium heat. Sauté the onion for 5 minutes, until soft, then add the garlic and cook for another minute. Add the red pepper and sauté for another 5 minutes, until tender. Stir in the paprika and cumin and cook for 1 minute. Stir in the tomatoes and season.

Place the tofu on top, cover with a lid, and simmer for 10 minutes. Remove the lid, transfer the casserole to the oven, and bake for 10 minutes, until the tofu has crisped. Divide between four plates and garnish with the parsley and avocado slices.

Flex it – *Replace the tofu with egg for a non-vegan version.*

Salmon teriyaki

Serves 4
Prep 5 mins
Cook 15–20 mins

**4x 150g (5¹/₂oz) salmon
 fillets
1 tbsp clear honey
2 tsp sesame oil
2 tbsp mirin
4 tbsp tamari soy sauce
4 tsp grated ginger
steamed tenderstem
 broccoli, asparagus,
 or bok choy, to serve**

Flex it *– To reduce the sugar,
use just ¹/₂ tbsp of honey and
¹/₂ tbsp of orange juice.*

**helps calm hot flushes • aids cognition
• promotes bone health**

This sweet salmon dish is high in omega-3, which,
together with soy and sesame, may ease hot flushes.
Sesame also provides calcium for healthy bones and
anti-inflammatory ginger supports brain health.

Preheat the oven to 200°C (425°F/Gas 7). Place the
salmon in a shallow baking dish.

In a bowl, mix together the honey, sesame oil, mirin,
tamari, and ginger, then pour evenly over the salmon,
ensuring it is well covered. Bake for 15–20 minutes,
or until the salmon is cooked and flakes easily with
a knife. Serve warm with steamed tenderstem broccoli,
asparagus, or bok choy, or eat cold as part of a salad.

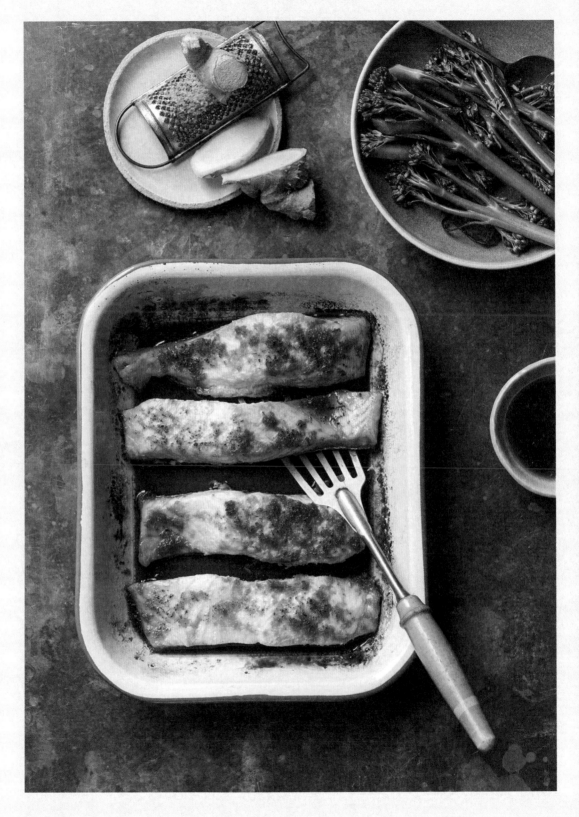

Salmon teriyaki

Kale, chicken, *and* Parmesan bowl

Serves 4
Prep 5 mins
Cook 25 mins

2 tbsp olive oil
400g (14oz) kale, stems
    removed and chopped
500g (1lb 2oz) skinless
    chicken breast, cut into
    smaller fillets
4 garlic cloves, thinly sliced
40g (1$^{1}/_{2}$oz) pine nuts, rinsed
juice of 1 lemon
140g (5oz) Parmesan,
    roughly grated

helps manage weight • aids sleep
• aids cognition

In this high-protein, filling bowl kale provides magnesium – key for nerve function and healthy cognition – while chicken supplies sleep-promoting tryptophan, helping to relieve menopausal fatigue.

Heat a large frying pan over a medium heat. Add half the olive oil and the kale and toss the kale for a few minutes until wilted. Remove from the pan and set aside.

Heat the remaining olive oil in the pan and add the chicken fillets. Stir until cooked through and golden brown. Remove and set aside.

Add the garlic and pine nuts to the pan and stir for 1–2 minutes, until golden brown. Return the kale and chicken to the pan and add the lemon juice and Parmesan. Toss to combine all the ingredients well and serve immediately.

Roasted Dijon chicken

Serves 4
Prep 5 mins
Cook 1 hour 35 mins
Rest 5 mins

2 tbsp olive oil
2 tbsp Dijon mustard
1 whole chicken, about 1.5kg
  (3lb 3oz)
1 lemon, quartered
1 garlic bulb, sliced at the top
roasted root vegetables, such
  as carrots, sweet potatoes,
  and parsnips, to serve

supports heart health • boosts immunity

Enjoying a whole chicken provides a range of immune-boosting nutrients, the darker flesh of the thighs being most nutrient dense. Olive oil contains oleic acid, to support healthy blood vessels.

Preheat the oven to 190°C (400°F/Gas 6). Place the olive oil and mustard in a small bowl and stir well to combine. Place the chicken in an ovenproof dish and cover it with the olive–mustard mixture. Place the lemon in the chicken cavity then cook in the oven for 20 minutes. Turn the chicken over and add the garlic. Peel and chop the root vegetables and add to the dish with the chicken. Baste the chicken in its juices and cook for another 20 minutes.

Turn the chicken over one last time, baste again, and cook for another 20–35 minutes, or until the juices run clear and you can easily detach the leg joints with a knife and fork. Serve with the roasted root vegetables.

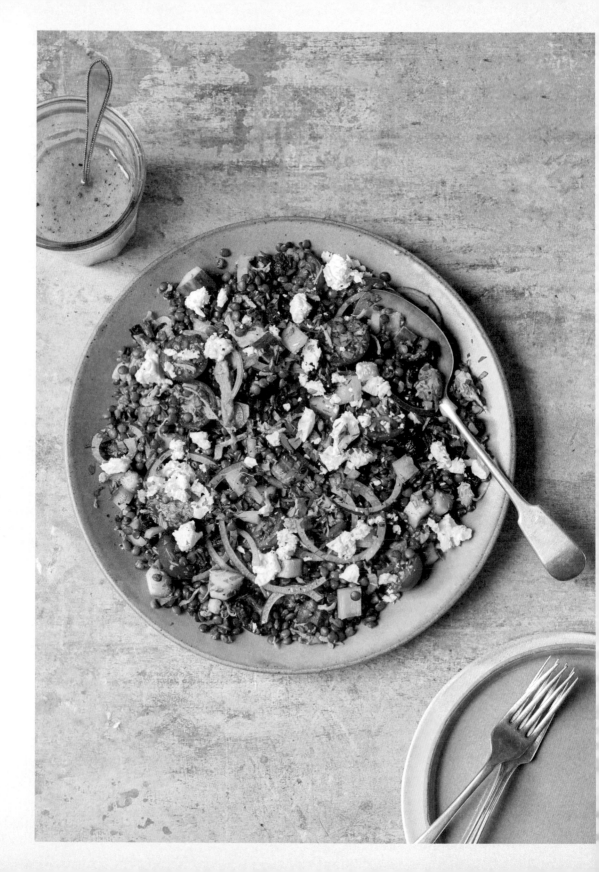

Puy lentils, ham, *and* feta salad

helps manage weight • supports heart health • provides sustained energy

This satiating salad is packed with iron and folate, two nutrients that are often low in the menopause transition. Vitamin C in the tomatoes and lemon supports iron absorption.

Serves 4
Prep 15 mins
Cook 15 mins
Rest 1–2 hours

300g (10oz) Puy lentils
100g (3¹/₂oz) cooked ham hock, shredded
100g (3¹/₂oz) feta, diced
1 small cucumber, diced
1 yellow pepper, deseeded and diced
12 cherry tomatoes, halved
1 red onion, thinly sliced
50g (1³/₄oz) black olives, pitted and halved
50g (1³/₄oz) sun-dried tomatoes
25g (scant 1oz) flat-leaf parsley, finely chopped

For the dressing
juice and zest of 2 lemons
3 tbsp olive oil
sea salt and freshly ground black pepper

Cook the lentils according to the packet instructions. Drain, cool, and set aside. To make the dressing, place the lemon juice and zest, olive oil, and salt and pepper in a bowl, stir, and set aside.

In a large serving bowl, add the lentils, dressing, and the remaining ingredients, then stir carefully to combine. Serve or refrigerate for 1–2 hours for the flavours to develop.

Flex it *– For a vegetarian option, remove the ham hock.*

Baked cod *with* lemon sauce

Serves 4
Prep 10 mins
Cook 10–15 mins

4x 150g (5¹/₂oz) cod fillets
sea salt and freshly
   ground black pepper
50g (1³/₄oz) butter or ghee
100g (3¹/₂oz) crème fraîche
2 garlic cloves, crushed
30g (1oz) Dijon mustard
2 tbsp lemon juice
flat-leaf parsley, to garnish
steamed new potatoes,
   wilted spinach, and
   lemon wedges, to serve

helps manage weight • provides sustained energy • supports muscle health

White fish is a good source of filling protein, satisfying the appetite and protecting against muscle loss in midlife.

Preheat the oven to 200°C (425°F/Gas 7). Place the cod in a baking dish, leaving some space in between the fillets. Season.

Place the butter or ghee, crème fraîche, garlic, mustard, and lemon juice in a small pan over a low heat. Stir to combine. As soon as the butter is melted and the mixture is smooth, pour over the fish. Bake for 10–15 minutes, or until the fish is just cooked and flakes easily with a knife. Serve immediately with the steamed new potatoes, spinach, and lemon wedges.

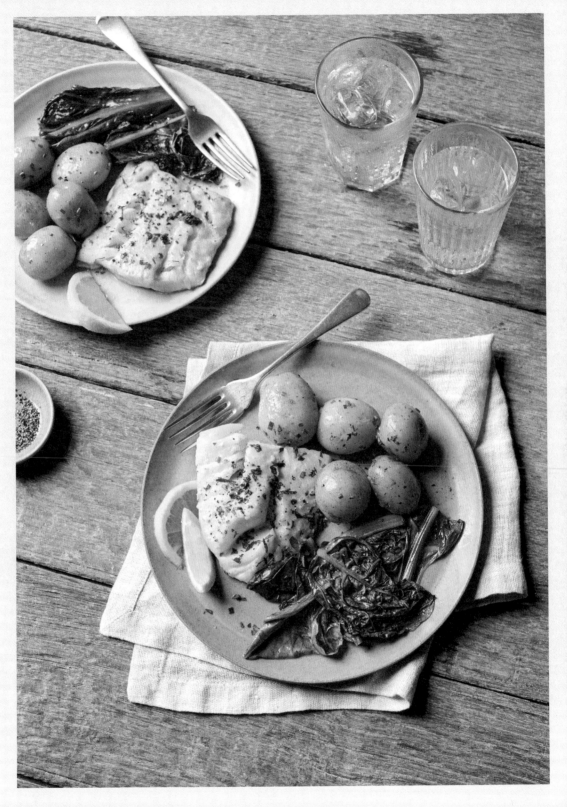

Baked cod with lemon sauce

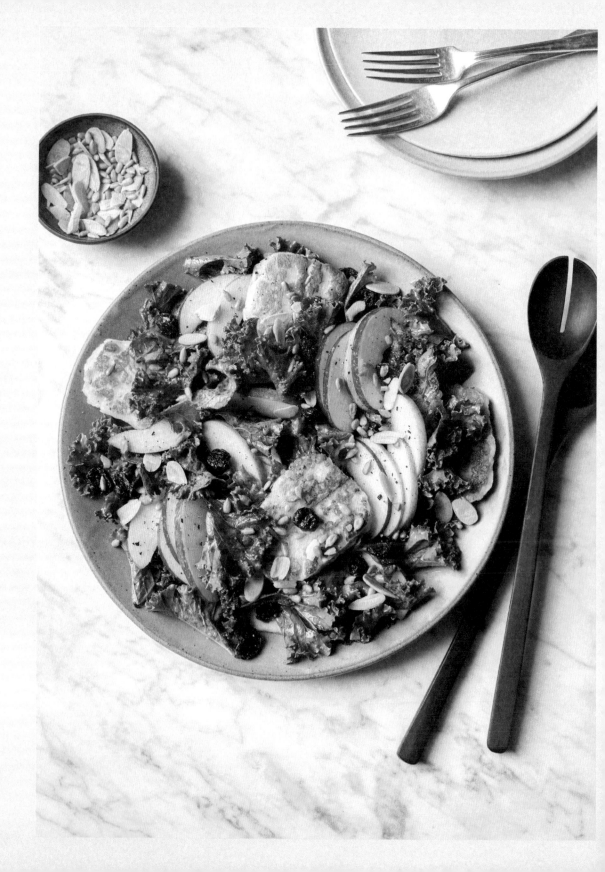

Magical kale salad

Serves 4
Prep 30 mins
Cook 7 mins
Rest 1–2 hours

200g (7oz) kale, stalks removed
1 apple, cored and thinly sliced
1 tbsp olive oil
200g (7oz) halloumi, sliced
juice of 1 lemon
50g (1³/₄oz) flaked almonds
50g (1³/₄oz) sunflower seeds
50g (1³/₄oz) dried cranberries
   or sultanas
sea salt flakes (optional)

For the dressing
1 apple, cored and roughly
   chopped
5cm (2in) piece of fresh root
   ginger, peeled and chopped
1 tbsp clear honey
3 tbsp tamari soy sauce
1 tbsp olive oil
1 tbsp sesame oil
2 tsp ground cinnamon
2 tsp sumac
juice of 1 lemon

Flex it – *Add egg to up the protein.*
For a vegan dish, swap the halloumi
with tempeh.

promotes bone health • supports heart health
• promotes healthy joints

Leafy green kale is rich in magnesium and calcium for bone health. Healthy fats in almonds, olive oil, and sunflower seeds support heart health; and ginger helps fight inflammation, protecting joints.

To make the dressing, blend all the ingredients in a food processor until smooth.

Put the kale and apple in a large salad bowl, pour over the dressing, and mix well, using your hands to wilt the leaves a little. Refrigerate for 1–2 hours to allow the flavours to develop.

In a pan, heat the olive oil on a medium heat, add the halloumi slices, and cook for 3 minutes; turn and cook for another 3 minutes. Once golden, add the lemon juice and after 30 seconds, turn again. Set aside.

Place the halloumi slices on top of the salad and sprinkle with the flaked almonds, sunflower seeds, dried cranberries, and, if desired, some sea salt flakes.

Three beans salad

Serves 4
Prep 15 mins
Rest 1 hour

**500g (1lb 2oz) red kidney
beans, cooked**
**500g (1lb 2oz) chickpeas,
cooked**
**400g (14oz) green beans,
cooked and cut into thirds**
1 red onion, finely diced
**25g (scant 1oz) flat-leaf
parsley, finely chopped**

For the dressing
**4 tbsp extra virgin
olive oil**
**3³/₄ tbsp raw apple cider
vinegar**
**1 tbsp wholegrain Dijon
mustard**
**sea salt and freshly ground
black pepper**

Flex it – *For extra protein,
add boiled eggs, crumbled feta,
mozzarella balls, or pan-fried
halloumi slices.*

**helps manage weight • supports digestion
• promotes bone health • supports muscle health**

This simple, but satisfying, salad is an excellent
source of plant proteins – for bone and muscle
strength – and fibre, aiding digestion and helping
to regulate your appetite between meals.

For the dressing, place all the ingredients in a small
bowl and stir well.

Place the dressing, all the beans, and the onion and
parsley in a large bowl and combine well. Refrigerate
for 1 hour before serving.

Roast leg of lamb

Serves 4
Prep 30 mins
Cook 1 hour 30 mins
Rest 10 mins

**1.5kg (3lb 3oz) leg of lamb,
    bone in**
4 garlic cloves, sliced
**2 sprigs of rosemary,
    leaves removed and
    roughly chopped**
olive oil
**sea salt and freshly
    ground black pepper**
**green beans and gratin
    potatoes, to serve**

**promotes muscle health • supports cognition
• helps manage weight**

Dense in filling protein, a good supply of which is vital in menopause, lamb also has omega-3 fatty acids to support brain health, and the amino acid creatine, which helps maintain muscle mass.

Preheat the oven to 200°C (450°F/Gas 8).

Place the lamb in a roasting pan. Cut 2cm ($^3/_4$in) slits in the flesh and place the garlic slices and rosemary in the slits. If the lamb has been refrigerated, bring it to room temperature.

Before cooking, drizzle the lamb with olive oil and season with salt and pepper. Roast the lamb for 15–20 minutes, then reduce the oven heat to 130°C (300°F/Gas 2) and roast for a further 20–25 minutes per 450g (1lb) for medium–rare, or for another 25–30 minutes per 450g (1lb) for medium.

Rest the lamb for 10–15 minutes, covered with the foil. Carve and serve with green beans and gratin potatoes.

(photographed overleaf)

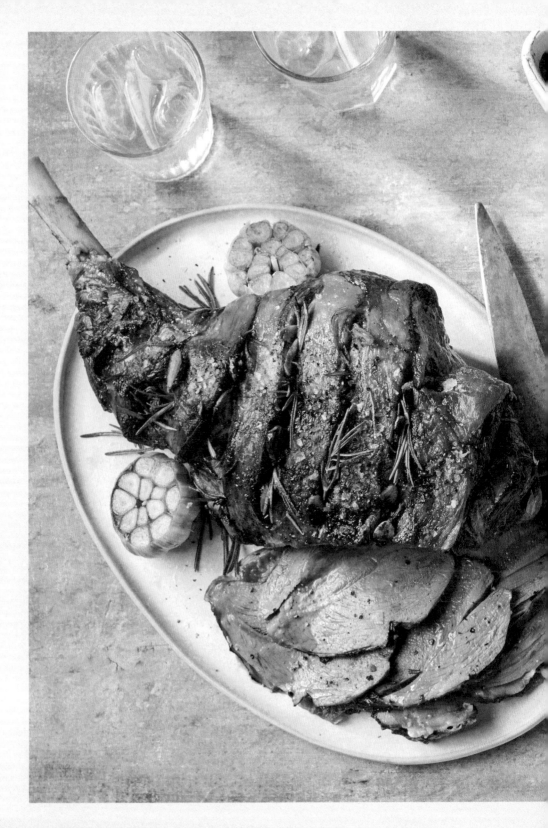

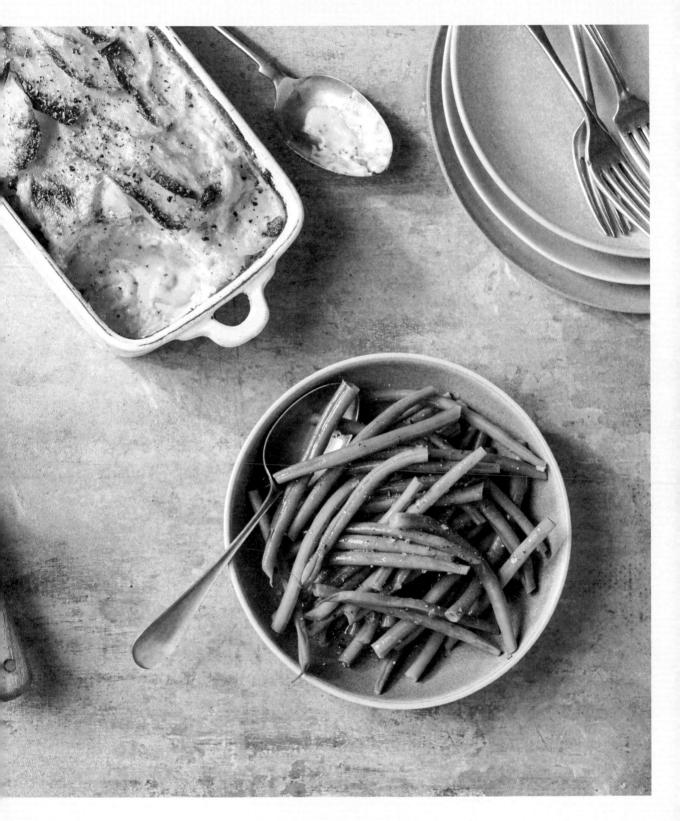

Roast leg of lamb

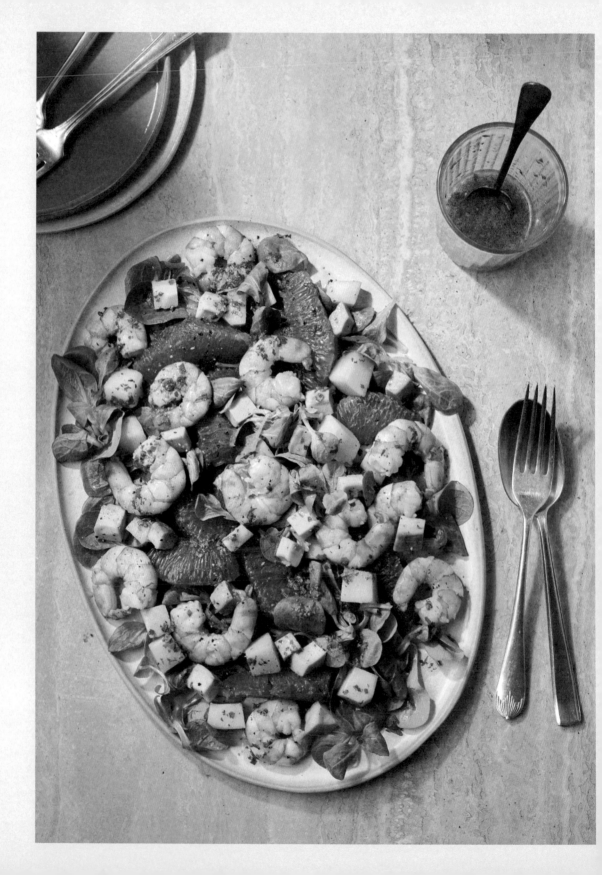

Prawn, avocado, grapefruit, *and* mango salad

promotes bone health • aids cognition • supports metabolism

Prawns provide a host of minerals, including selenium, zinc, and iron, vital for thyroid health, while mango supplies antioxidant beta-carotene, promoting healthy brain function. If taking medication, check with your doctor before eating grapefruit.

Serves 4
Prep 20 mins
Rest 1 hour (optional)

2 avocados, pitted and diced
juice of 1 lime
600g (1lb 5oz) cooked prawns,
   peeled and deveined
2 grapefruits, segments
   separated and pith removed

1 mango, diced
400g (14oz) lamb's lettuce

For the dressing
4 tbsp lemon juice
4 tbsp extra virgin
   olive oil
1 tsp Dijon mustard
10g (¼oz) coriander,
   finely chopped

Place the avocado in a serving bowl, add the lime juice, and stir gently to coat the avocado and prevent it from browning. Add the remaining salad ingredients and set aside.

Place all the dressing ingredients in a bowl, stir well, and add to the serving bowl. Carefully combine the salad and dressing. If you wish, refrigerate for 1 hour to enhance the flavours before serving.

Flex it – *For extra protein, grate some Parmesan over, or add small mozzarella balls to the salad.*

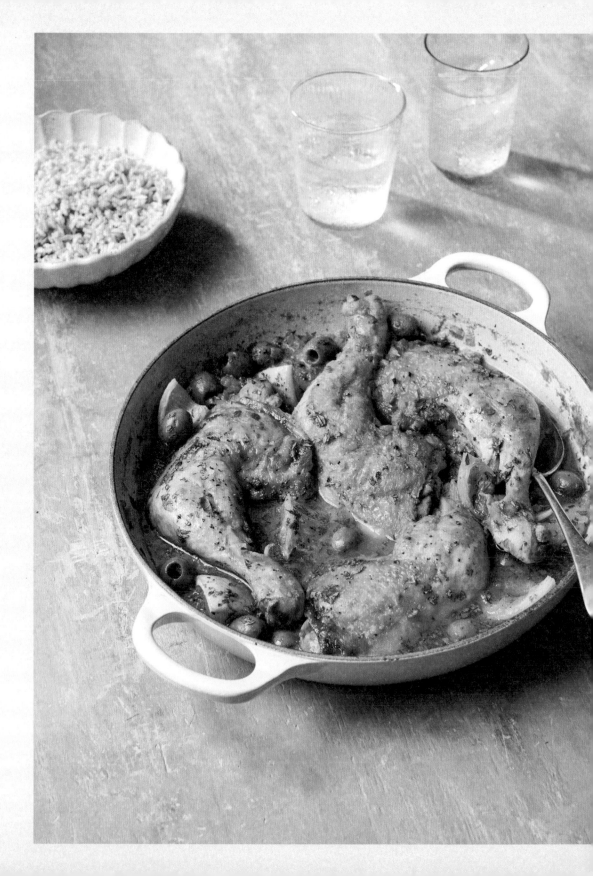

Chicken *with* green olives

calms • aids sleep • boosts immunity

Darker cuts of chicken yield the most immune-supporting micronutrients. A chicken supper can aid sleep as it contains the amino acid tryptophan, a precursor to sleep-promoting serotonin and melatonin.

Serves 4
Prep 5 mins
Cook 1 hour

3 tbsp olive oil
4 chicken legs (thighs and
    drumsticks)
1 onion, finely chopped
3 garlic cloves, sliced
1 tsp ground ginger
1 tsp ground turmeric

500ml (16fl oz) chicken bone
    broth (see p.216)
25g (scant 1oz) coriander,
    chopped
25g (scant 1oz) flat-leaf parsley,
    chopped
100g (3½oz) green olives, pitted
1 lemon, cut into 8 parts
sea salt and freshly ground
    black pepper
basmati rice or quinoa, to serve

Heat a flameproof casserole over a medium heat, add the olive oil, and brown the chicken. Remove and set aside.

Add the onion and cook until translucent, about 5 minutes. Add the garlic and spices and cook for another 3–5 minutes, stirring to ensure that the spices do not burn. Return the chicken to the casserole, add the bone broth, and bring to the boil. Add the herbs, olives, lemon, and seasoning. Combine well, then simmer for about 45 minutes, until the meat detaches easily. Serve with basmati rice or quinoa.

Savoury crêpes

Makes 6–8 crêpes
Prep 5 mins
Cook 5–7 mins per crêpe

For the batter
2 eggs
100g (3¹/₂oz) buckwheat flour
400ml (14fl oz) unsweetened milk of your choice

Filling suggestions per person
¹/₂–1 slice of ham and 30g (1oz) grated Cheddar
1 egg and 30g (1oz) grated Cheddar
¹/₂–1 slice of ham, 1 egg, and 30g (1oz) grated Cheddar
50g (1³/₄oz) cooked mushrooms, ¹/₄ cooked onion, and rosemary
40g (1¹/₂oz) cooked spinach and 30g (1oz) goat's cheese
40g (1¹/₂oz) cooked leeks and 1 egg
40g (1¹/₂oz) cooked spinach and 1 slice smoked salmon

knob of butter or ghee (optional)
green side salad, to serve

helps manage weight • balances moods • boosts immunity

Taking minutes to prep, these delicious crêpes are a protein-rich sustaining meal that steadies blood sugars, removing the urge to snack. Add spinach to any combo for an antioxidant immunity boost.

To make the batter, place all the ingredients in a food processor and blend until smooth.

Heat a 23cm (9in) pancake pan on a medium heat. If you wish, add a knob of butter or ghee and tilt the pan to swirl it, so that the butter coats the surface evenly. Adding butter or ghee helps the first pancake to not stick and adds colour and a richer flavour.

Carefully add a ladle – about 100ml (3¹/₂fl oz) – of the mixture to the pan. Tilt the pan to swirl the batter and coat the surface evenly. Cook for about 2 minutes, until the batter bubbles and the base is light brown. Loosen with a silicon spatula, turn, and cook the other side.

As soon as you turn the pancake, add the filling then fold in each side of the pancake. Cook for 2 minutes, turn again, and cook for another 2 minutes. Serve warm with a green side salad.

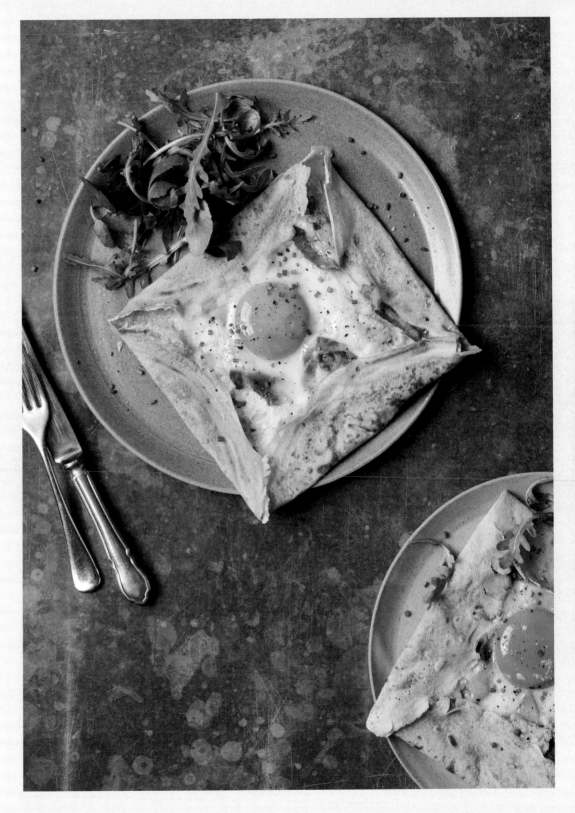

Savoury crêpes

Beef *and* liver meatballs

helps balance hormones • supports heart health

This combo marries protein-dense beef with nutrient-dense liver, both of which provide easily absorbed iron. It also has saturated fat, a source of cholesterol, needed for the production of the hormones oestrogen, progesterone, and testosterone.

Makes 3 balls per serving
Prep 15 mins
Cook 25–30 mins

150g (5½oz) chicken liver, finely diced
450g (1lb) minced beef
1 onion, finely diced
¼ tsp sea salt
60g (2oz) Parmesan, grated
2 eggs
wholegrain or wild rice and tenderstem broccoli, to serve

Preheat the oven to 190°C (400°F/Gas 6). Line a tray with parchment paper. Place all the ingredients in a large bowl and mix with your hands until well combined.

Wet your clean hands and form 12 balls, around 50g (1¾oz) each, placing each meatball on the tray. Bake for 25–30 minutes, or until the meatballs are cooked through. Serve warm with wholegrain or wild rice and tenderstem broccoli.

Liver, onion, *and* sage

aids cognition • boosts immunity

Liver is one of the most nutritious foods, high in vitamin A for healthy skin and hair, B vitamins and choline, vital for brain health, and vitamin C for strengthened immunity.

Serves 4
Prep 10 mins
Cook 10 mins

6 tbsp olive oil
1 onion, finely sliced
40g (1½oz) buckwheat flour
1 tsp sea salt

400g (14oz) chicken liver, sliced
   into 3 strips
25g (scant 1oz) sage leaves,
   finely sliced
broccoli with rice, quinoa,
   or roasted sweet potatoes,
   to serve

In a large frying pan, heat 1 tablespoon of the olive oil on a medium heat. Add the onion and cook until translucent and tender, about 5 minutes. Remove from the pan and set aside.

Place the flour and salt in a bowl and combine. Add the liver and toss until well coated. Heat the remaining oil in the pan over a medium heat, add the strips of liver, and cook for a few minutes, flipping them halfway through – they should still be pink in the centre.

Return the onions to the pan and add the sage. Stir for a few minutes more. Serve immediately with broccoli and rice, quinoa, or starchy vegetables such as roasted sweet potatoes.

Pulled pork

Serves 8
Prep 5 mins
Cook 7–8 hours
Rest 30 mins

1.6kg (3lb 6oz) boneless pork shoulder, with fat
1 tbsp smoked paprika
2 tbsp brown sugar
2 tbsp salt
cucumber, apple cider, and dill salad or red cabbage, to serve

helps balance hormones • supports heart health • promotes muscle health

High in protein and nutrients, pork also provides cholesterol for hormone production, as well as the amino acids creatine, which promotes muscle strength, and taurine, for heart health.

Preheat the oven to 220°C (475°F/Gas 9). Place a large piece of foil in a roasting tin and place the pork in the tin, fat side up.

Combine the paprika, sugar, and salt in a small bowl and rub the mixture over the pork. Cook the pork for about 40 minutes, then reduce the heat to 120°C (300°F/Gas 2), fold the foil around the pork and cook for a further 6–7 hours, until the pork detaches easily with a fork.

Return the heat to 220°C (475°F/Gas 9) and cook, uncovered, for another 10 minutes. Rest for 30 minutes, then shred the pork and serve immediately with a cucumber, apple cider, and dill salad, or with red cabbage.

Orange *and* herb-roasted turkey breast

Serves 4
Prep 10 mins
Cook 40 mins
Rest 5 mins

2 oranges, each cut into
    8 pieces
sea salt and freshly ground
    black pepper
1 turkey breast, about 600g
    (1lb 5oz)
2 tbsp olive oil
2 tbsp sage, finely chopped
2 tbsp rosemary, finely
    chopped
2 tbsp thyme, finely chopped
rainbow salsa (p.171),
    to serve

**aids sleep • helps calm hot flushes
• aids memory**

Turkey has sleep-supporting tryptophan, and is a source of B vitamins, key for energy, cognition, and stress. Adding flavoursome sage helps ease hot flushes. Chicken can be used instead of turkey here.

Preheat the oven to 200°C (425°F/Gas 7). Arrange the orange pieces in a roasting tin. Season the turkey breast with salt and pepper and place it on top of the oranges.

Place the olive oil and herbs in a bowl and combine well. Spoon the herb mixture evenly over the turkey. Add 1 cup of water to the bottom of the roasting tin, to cover the oranges but not the bottom of the turkey. Bake for 30–40 minutes, until the meat is cooked and the skin is brown and crisp. Check the water level during baking and add more if it evaporates too quickly, to prevent the oranges from burning.

Discard the oranges. Leave the turkey breast to rest for a few minutes at room temperature before slicing. Serve the turkey with the rainbow salsa on page 171.

Sweet potato, kale, *and* sausage bowl

Serves 4
Prep 20 mins
Cook 45 mins

300g (10oz) sweet potato, peeled and diced
4 tbsp olive oil
sea salt and freshly ground black pepper
8 sausages, approximately 70g (2½oz) each, cut into 1.5cm (½in) slices
400g (14oz) kale, stalks removed
2 apples, peeled, cored, and sliced
coriander or flat-leaf parsley, to garnish

Flex it – *For a vegetarian option, try swapping the sausage for tempeh.*

boosts immunity • supports metabolism • balances hormones

This simple but varied dish marries protein and sweet potato – high in protective antioxidants – with cruciferous kale, which supports liver metabolism, in turn helping to balance hormones.

Preheat the oven to 190°C (400°F/Gas 6). Place the sweet potato on a baking tray, add half the olive oil, season, and stir to combine. Bake for 30 minutes, or until the potatoes are tender. Set aside.

Heat a frying pan on a medium heat, add the remaining olive oil and the sausages, and fry, stirring regularly, until the sausages are cooked. Remove and set aside.

Add the kale to the pan and stir for a few minutes until almost wilted. Add the sweet potatoes, sausages, and apples and stir for a few minutes to allow the flavours to combine. Serve warm, garnished with some coriander or parsley.

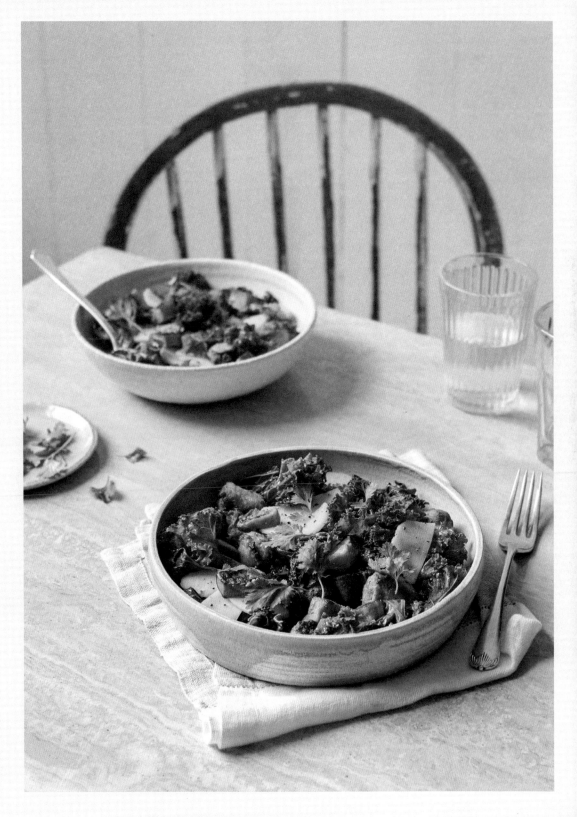

Sweet potato, kale, and sausage bowl

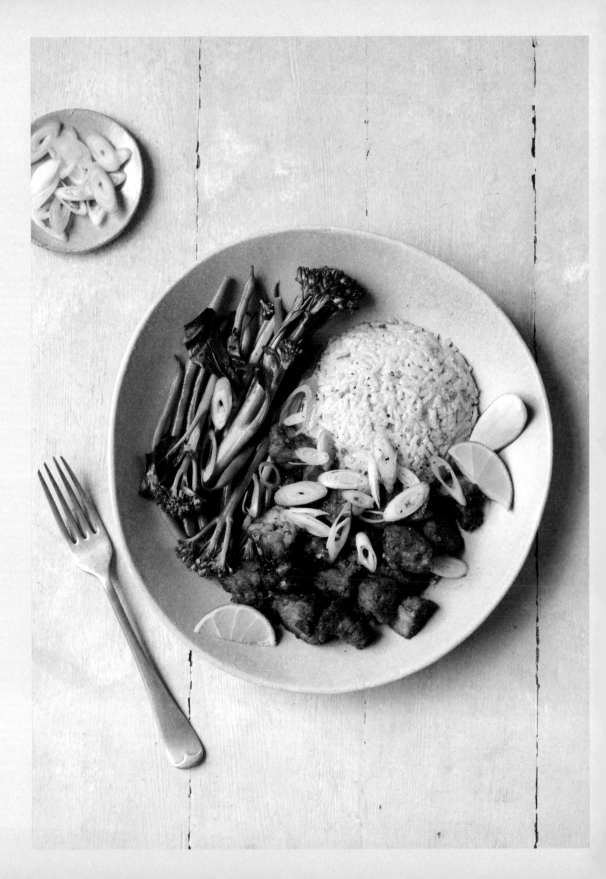

Sticky ginger tempeh *with* coconut rice

Serves 4
Prep 10 mins
Cook 35 mins

For the coconut rice
400ml can full-fat coconut milk
15g ($\frac{1}{2}$oz) coconut sugar
sea salt, to taste
100g ($3\frac{1}{2}$oz) basmati rice,
**   thoroughly rinsed**
$\frac{1}{2}$ tsp lime zest and 1 tsp
**   lime juice**

For the tempeh
400g (14oz) tempeh, pat dried
**   and diced**
120ml (4fl oz) tamari soy sauce
30g (1oz) coconut sugar
1 tsp lime juice
1 tbsp avocado oil
5cm (2in) piece of ginger,
**   peeled and finely chopped**
1 garlic clove, finely chopped
sea salt and freshly ground
**   black pepper**
2 spring onions, finely sliced,
**   to garnish**
steamed broccoli or green
**   beans and lime slices, to**
**   serve (optional)**

helps calm hot flushes • promotes gut health

This delicious vegan dish has phytoestrogens from the tempeh and tamari, while prebiotic spring onions, part of the allium family, support gut health.

For the rice, place the milk, 250ml (9fl oz) water, coconut sugar, and salt in a lidded pan over a high heat. Bring to the boil, stirring occasionally. Add the rice, stir, and return to the boil. Cover and simmer until almost all of the liquid is absorbed, about 15 minutes. Add the lime zest and juice and fluff the rice lightly. Cover to keep warm.

For the tempeh, add water to cover the base of a lidded frying pan. Bring to a simmer, add the tempeh, cover, and cook for 10 minutes. Remove the tempeh and set aside to cool. In a bowl, whisk the tamari, sugar, and lime juice.

Heat the oil over a medium heat in the cleaned pan. Add the tempeh and stir until lightly browned. Add the ginger and garlic and stir for 30 seconds, until fragrant. Add the tamari mix, stir, and cook for 6–7 minutes, until the sauce has caramelized slightly. Season. Serve immediately with the rice, spring onions, and lime slices. If desired, add steamed broccoli or green beans.

Beetroot *and* goat's cheese salad

Serves 4
Prep 20 mins

For the dressing
2 tbsp extra virgin olive oil
2 tbsp lemon juice
2 tsp Dijon mustard

400g (14oz) watercress
8 eggs, boiled, peeled, and halved
4 beetroot, cooked and diced
200g (7oz) goat's cheese, crumbled
50g (1³/₄oz) walnuts, roughly chopped
2 tbsp flat-leaf parsley, chopped

Flex it – *Add cooked chickpeas for extra protein.*

supports heart health • aids cognition • boosts immunity

This summer salad has solid benefits. Beetroot contains nitrates, boosting blood vessel health; omega-3s in walnuts aid brain function; and vitamin C-rich watercress supports immunity.

Place all the dressing ingredients in a bowl and blend together.

Place the salad ingredients, apart from the eggs and a little of the parsley, in a serving bowl. Pour over the dressing and combine gently, so that the beetroot doesn't colour the cheese. Layer the egg halves on top and scatter over the remaining parsley to serve.

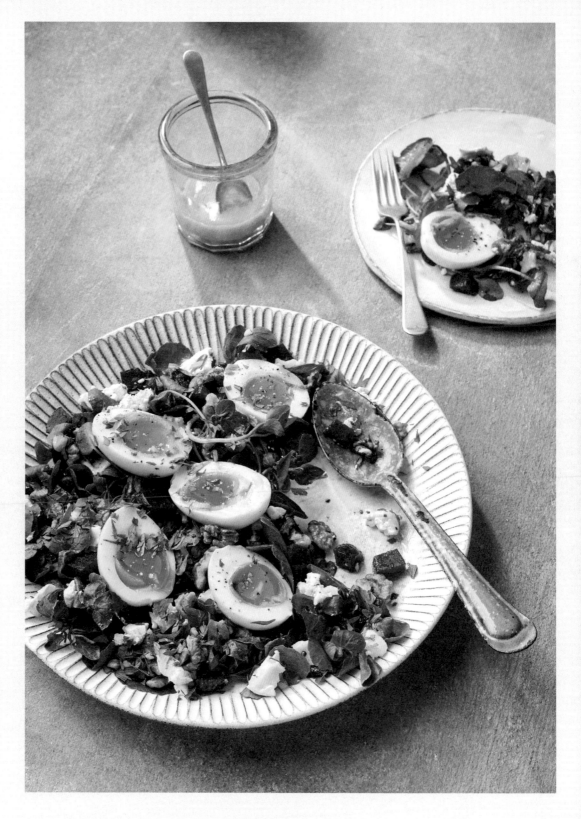

Beetroot and goat's cheese salad

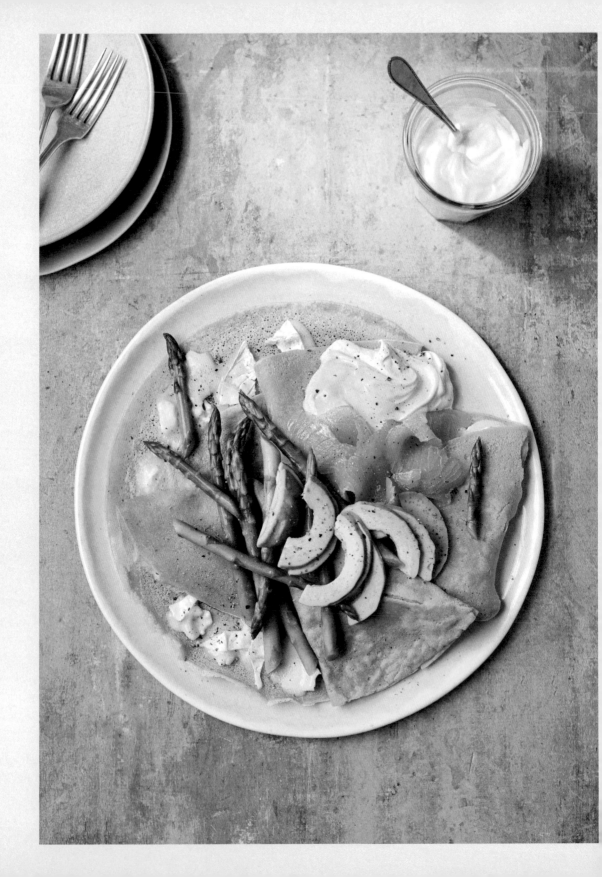

Chickpea crêpe *with* goat's cheese *and* asparagus

helps calm hot flushes • supports metabolism • balances hormones

Chickpeas are rich in plant-based protein, while turmeric supports liver function, aiding hormone metabolism to ease symptoms such as hot flushes.

Serves 4
Prep 5 mins
Cook 10 mins

240g (8¹/₂oz) chickpea (gram) flour
2 tsp turmeric
1 tsp sea salt
2 tsp olive oil
80g (3oz) goat's cheese

To serve
asparagus, steamed
2 avocados, pitted and sliced
4 slices of smoked salmon
crème fraîche, to serve

Prepare one crêpe at a time: blend together 60g (2oz) chickpea flour, 120ml (4fl oz) water, ¹/₂ teaspoon turmeric, and ¹/₄ teaspoon salt.

Heat a frying pan over a medium heat, add ¹/₂ teaspoon of the olive oil, then pour the mixture in and swirl it around to make sure it covers the pan evenly. Cook for 3–4 minutes, then turn.

Add a quarter of the goat's cheese to one half of the crêpe and let this melt. Once the crêpe is cooked on both sides, fold it over the cheese. Serve with asparagus, avocado slices, smoked salmon, and a dollop of crème fraîche on the side.

Crustless broccoli quiche

aids sleep • balances hormones • helps manage weight

This light quiche is high in sustaining protein. Broccoli supports liver metabolism, to help stabilize hormones, while dairy contains the sleep-supporting amino acid tryptophan, making this an ideal supper to promote restful sleep.

Serves 4
Prep 10–15 mins
Cook 30 mins

200g (7oz) broccoli, steamed
   and cut into small florets

4 eggs
200g (7oz) crème fraîche
100g (3¹/₂oz) Cheddar, grated
sea salt and freshly ground
   black pepper
green side salad, to serve

Preheat the oven to 190°C (400°F/Gas 6). Line a 23cm (9in) round oven tin with parchment paper. Scatter the broccoli into the tin.

In a large bowl, whisk the eggs, crème fraîche, and Cheddar. Season. Pour the mixture over the broccoli. Bang the tin once on the tabletop to remove any bubbles and bake in the oven for 30 minutes. Enjoy warm or cold with a green side salad to serve.

Flex it – *For extra protein, add to or replace the broccoli with cooked shredded chicken, or cooked diced bacon.*

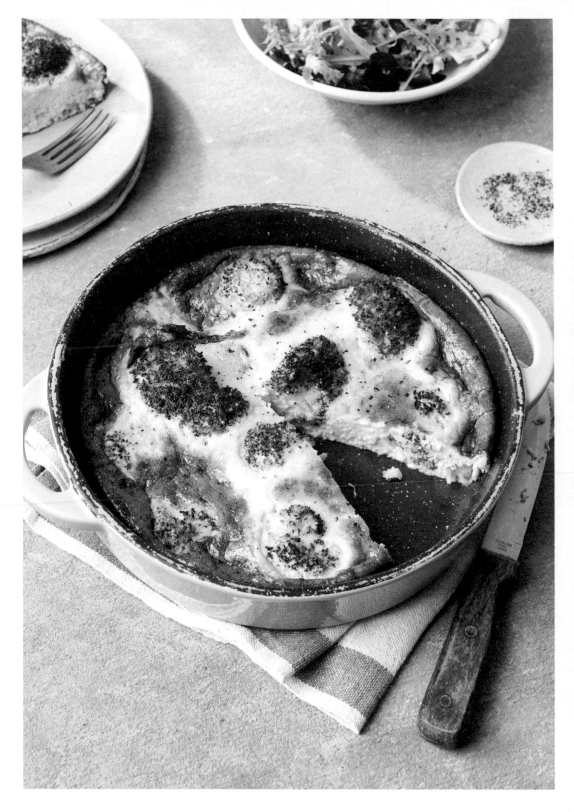

Crustless broccoli quiche

Tuna, salmon, *and* mackerel carpaccio

Serves 4
Prep 50 mins
Rest 2 hours

250g (9oz) tuna steak fillet
250g (9oz) mackerel fillet
250g (9oz) salmon fillet
3$\frac{1}{2}$ tbsp lime juice
100ml (3$\frac{1}{2}$fl oz) lemon juice
3$\frac{1}{2}$ tbsp extra virgin
   olive oil
15g ($\frac{1}{2}$oz) fresh ginger,
   grated
2$\frac{1}{2}$ tbsp tamari soy sauce
$\frac{1}{2}$ small fennel, finely diced
1 tsp dill, finely chopped
$\frac{1}{2}$ small red onion, finely
   sliced
1 tbsp small capers
wakame seaweed salad and
   rainbow salsa (p.171),
   to serve

**energizes • aids cognition
• has anti-inflammatory properties**

This filling dish is bursting with omega-3 fatty acids, helping to lift mood, support brain health, and control inflammation. It is also full of protein for healthy muscles and hormone production.

Wrap each fish fillet in cling film and freeze for 24 hours. Take out of the freezer, remove the cling film, and leave at room temperature for a few minutes, then carefully slice each fillet as thinly as possible with a very sharp knife. Place each fillet in a separate dish, or arrange them separately in one dish.

Drizzle the tuna with the lime juice, the salmon with the lemon juice, and the mackerel with the olive oil. Refrigerate for 1 hour.

In the meantime, mix the ginger and tamari in a small bowl. Once the fillets are ready to serve, top the tuna with the ginger and tamari; the mackerel with the fennel and dill; and the salmon with the red onion and capers. Serve with a wakame seaweed salad and the rainbow salsa on page 171.

Mains

146

Tofu *and* broccoli salad *with* peanut dressing

Serves 4
Prep 10 mins
Cook 25–30 mins

2 tbsp tamari soy sauce
2 tbsp rice vinegar
1½ tbsp sesame oil
400g (14oz) firm tofu,
sliced or diced
50g (1¾oz) peanut butter
500g (1lb 2oz) broccoli,
chopped into tiny florets
250g (9oz) radishes, finely
sliced
50g (1¾oz) raw peanuts,
roasted

Flex it – *Replace the tofu with*
500g (1lb 2oz) chicken for a
meaty version of this dish.

helps calm hot flushes • provides sustained energy • supports digestion

Phytoestrogenic tofu, nuts, broccoli, and radishes provide a complete meal, with omega-6 fats, protein, and healthy carbs and fibre.

Preheat the oven to 200°C (425°F/Gas 7). Line a baking sheet with parchment paper. In a flat dish, mix together half each of the tamari, rice vinegar, and sesame oil. Add the tofu and marinate for 15 minutes, flipping a couple of times.

Place the tofu on the baking sheet, spacing the pieces out. Bake for 25–30 minutes, turning halfway through.

In the meantime, place the peanut butter and 1–2 tablespoons of water in a bowl along with the remaining tamari, rice vinegar, and sesame oil and combine well.

Place the broccoli and radishes in a salad bowl, add the peanut dressing, and toss to combine. Top with the crispy tofu and peanuts to serve.

(photographed overleaf)

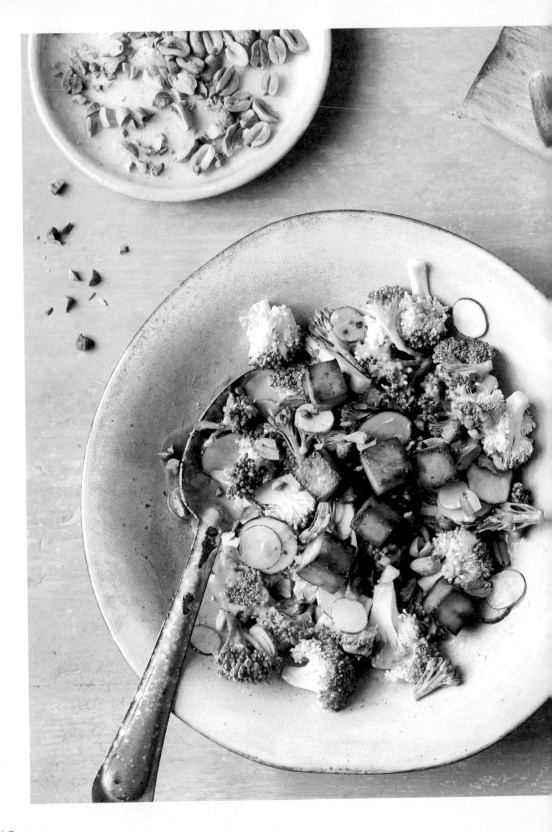

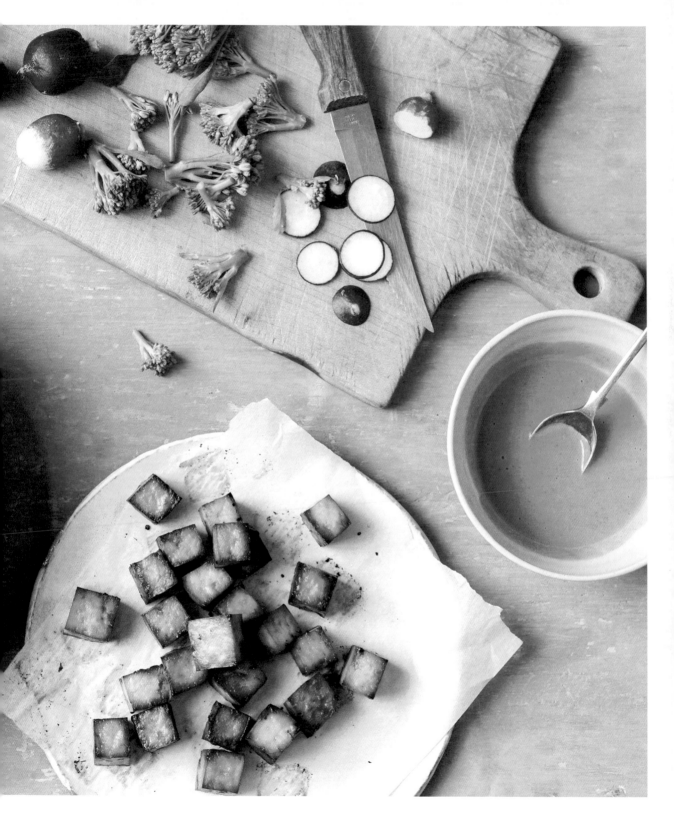

Tofu and broccoli salad with peanut dressing

Rainbow tempeh bowls

Serves 4
Prep 10–15 mins
Cook 30 mins

200g (7oz) brown rice
1 head of broccoli, chopped
    into florets
2 tbsp olive oil
2 tsp sesame oil
75ml (2½fl oz) tamari soy
    sauce
juice of 2 limes
1 garlic clove, crushed
1 tbsp clear honey or maple
    syrup
80g (3oz) smooth peanut
    butter
pinch of sea salt
400g (14oz) tempeh, diced
2 avocados, pitted and
    sliced
4 large carrots, peeled and
    julienned
16 cherry tomatoes, halved
½ small purple cabbage,
    thinly sliced
2 tbsp coriander, finely
    chopped
2 tbsp sesame seeds,
    roasted

helps calm hot flushes • supports digestion

This colourful vegan dish is high in antioxidants and healthy fats. Tempeh – fermented soy – is dense in isoflavones, to ease hot flushes, and fibre-rich brown rice supports bowel function.

Cook the rice according to the packet instructions. Preheat the oven to 200°C (425°F/Gas 7). Place the broccoli and olive oil in a bowl, toss to combine, then place on a baking sheet lined with parchment paper. Bake for 20 minutes, or until tender but not burned. Remove and set aside.

In a blender, add half the sesame oil, half the tamari, half the lime juice, the garlic, honey or maple syrup, peanut butter, and salt, and blend until smooth. Add 1 tablespoon of water to thin if needed. Refrigerate.

Place the remaining sesame oil, tamari, and lime juice in a bowl and stir well. Add the tempeh and toss to combine. Leave to marinate for 5 minutes. Heat a pan over a medium heat and add the tempeh. Cook for 5–7 minutes, stirring regularly. Remove and set aside.

Divide the rice, broccoli, avocado, carrots, tomatoes, purple cabbage, and tempeh evenly between four serving bowls. Drizzle over the peanut sauce. Sprinkle with the coriander, followed by the sesame seeds.

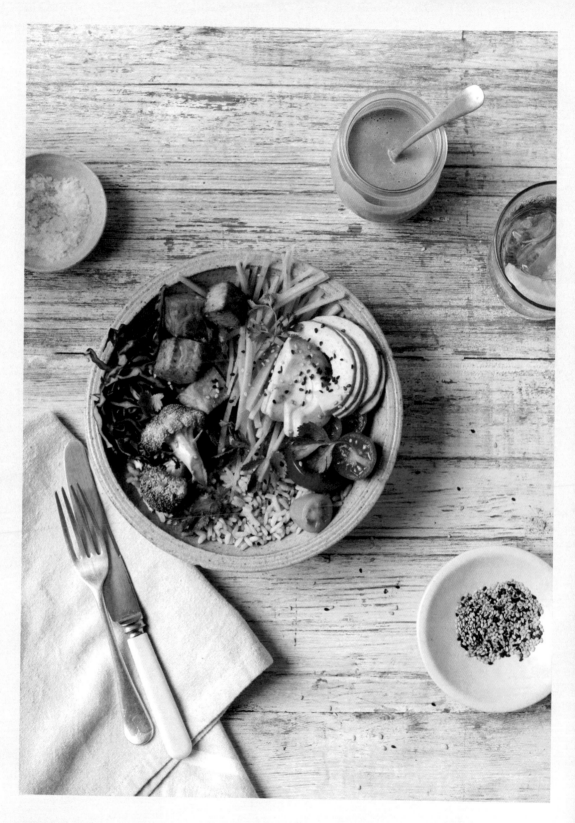

Rainbow tempeh bowls

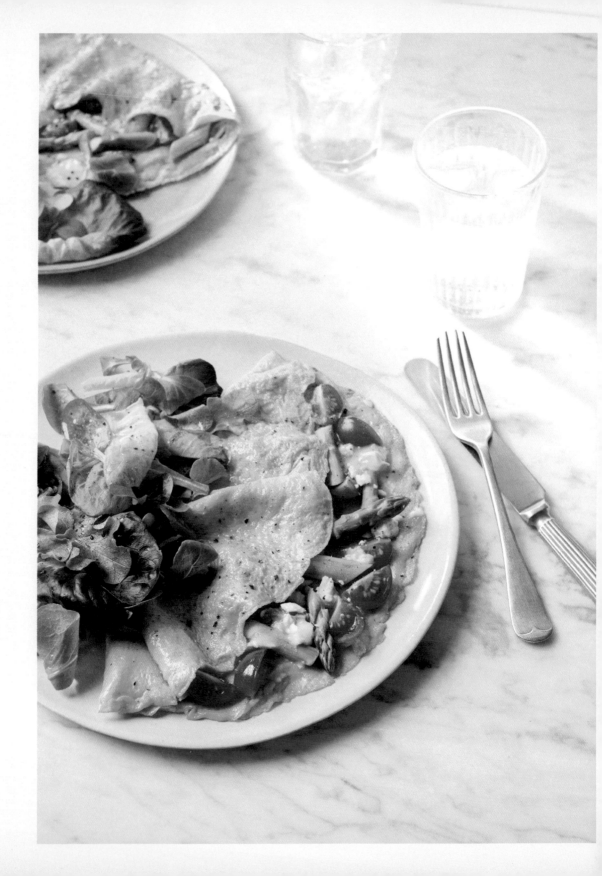

Omelette *with a* selection *of* fillings

promotes bone health • helps manage weight

Quick to rustle up, these omelettes are an easy way to boost protein levels, keeping you full and supporting bone health.

Serves 4
Prep 5–10 mins
Cook 5 mins

2 tbsp olive oil
8–12 eggs, beaten
herbs of choice (optional)
green side salad, to serve
  (optional)

Filling suggestions per person
1 slice of ham and 35g (1¼oz)
  grated cheese

½ tomato, diced, 2 cooked
  asparagus spears, cut into 2cm
  (¾in) pieces, and 35g (1¼oz)
  goat's cheese, crumbled
a handful of spinach and
  35g (1¼oz) goat's cheese
40g (1½oz) bacon, cooked and
  diced, and ½ tomato, diced
25g (scant 1oz) chives or any
  fresh herb, chopped
a handful of mushrooms or
  other vegetables, cooked

Ideally, prepare one omelette at a time, or one for two people if you have a large frying pan, using two to three eggs per person. Heat a frying pan over a medium heat and add the olive oil. If using herbs, beat the egg with the herbs.

Pour the egg into the pan and tilt the pan slightly from side to side, to cover the surface of the pan. Add your chosen filling.

Cook for 20–30 seconds, then score through the egg a couple of times so the uncooked runny egg fills the gaps. Do this until the egg has just set. Fold the omelette and serve immediately with a green side salad, if desired.

Baked eggs *with* spinach, tomato, *and* feta

Serves 4
Prep 15 mins
Cook 15–20 mins

300g (10oz) new potatoes,
  boiled and cut into
  chunks
300g (10oz) baby spinach,
  washed, wilted, and all
  water squeezed out
400ml (14fl oz) passata
1 garlic clove, thinly
  sliced
sea salt and freshly
  ground black pepper
4 eggs
1 tsp paprika
200g (7oz) feta cheese,
  crumbled

helps manage weight • provides sustained energy • supports bone health

Potatoes, spinach, and feta make a satisfying, flavoursome meal. Leafy green spinach provides magnesium and calcium for bones, and iron, whose absorption is aided by the vitamin C-rich passata.

Preheat the oven to 200°C (425°F/Gas 7). Place the potatoes at the bottom of an ovenproof dish. Scatter over the spinach then add the passata. Sprinkle over half the garlic and season with the salt and pepper.

Make four evenly spaced wells in the dish and crack an egg into each well. Sprinkle over the paprika, the remaining garlic, and dot over the feta. Bake for 15–20 minutes, until the eggs are cooked. Serve warm.

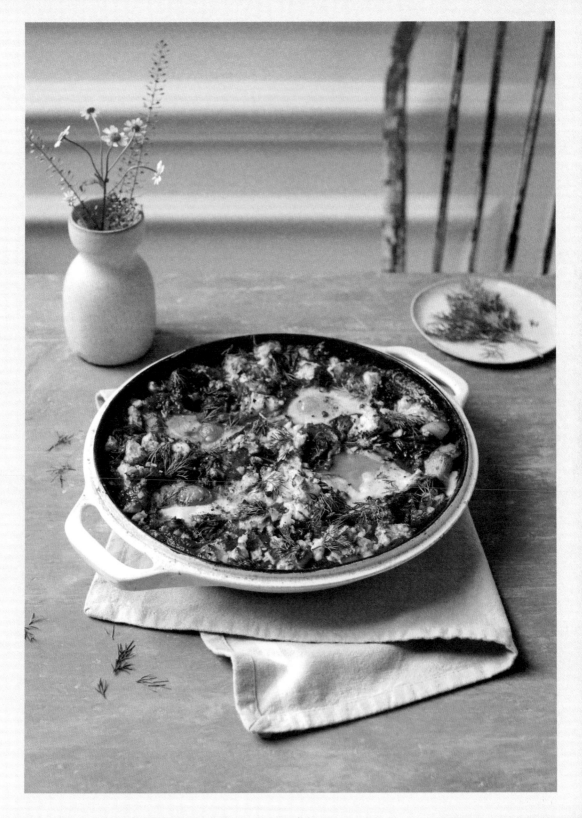

Baked eggs with spinach, tomatoes, and feta

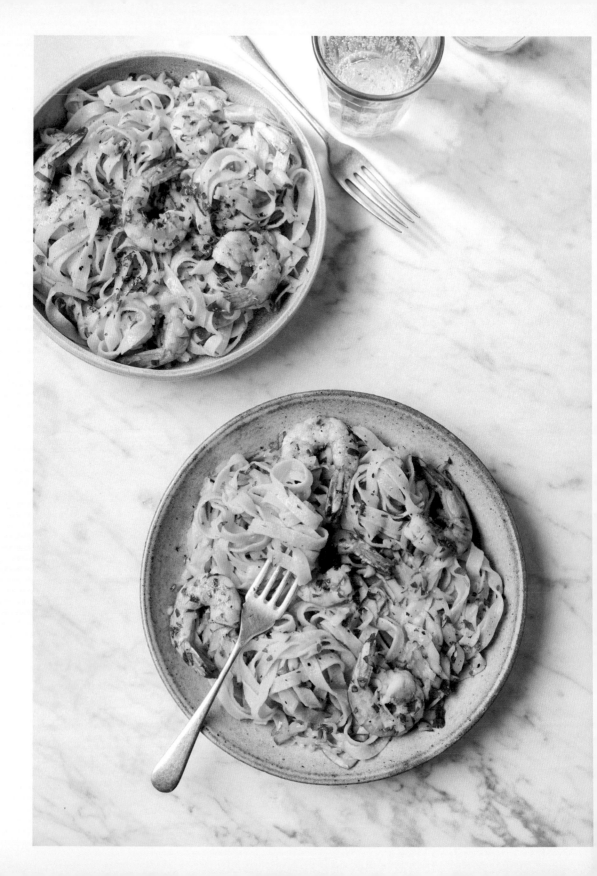

Courgette *and* prawn tagliatelle

energizes • helps hydrate • supports digestion • boosts immunity

Mineral-rich prawns are paired with hydrating courgettes here. Courgettes have a high water content to keep you energized and are also a source of fibre and immune-supporting vitamin C.

Serves 4
Prep 10 mins
Cook 10 mins

360g (12¹/₂oz) dried tagliatelle
4 tbsp olive oil
4 large courgettes, about 1kg (2¹/₄lb), peeled and coarsely grated

4 garlic cloves, finely grated
300g (10oz) raw king prawns, peeled and deveined
sea salt and freshly ground black pepper
zest and juice of 2 lemons
20g (³/₄oz) flat-leaf parsley, finely chopped

Cook the tagliatelle according to the packet instructions. In the meantime, heat a frying pan over a medium heat, add the olive oil, and fry the courgettes for about 4 minutes. Add the garlic, and cook for another 2 minutes. Add the prawns, season, and cook for a few minutes more, until pink.

Drain the tagliatelle, add it to the courgette and prawn mixture, and toss. Add the lemon zest and juice and stir to combine, then scatter over the parsley. Serve immediately.

Light bites

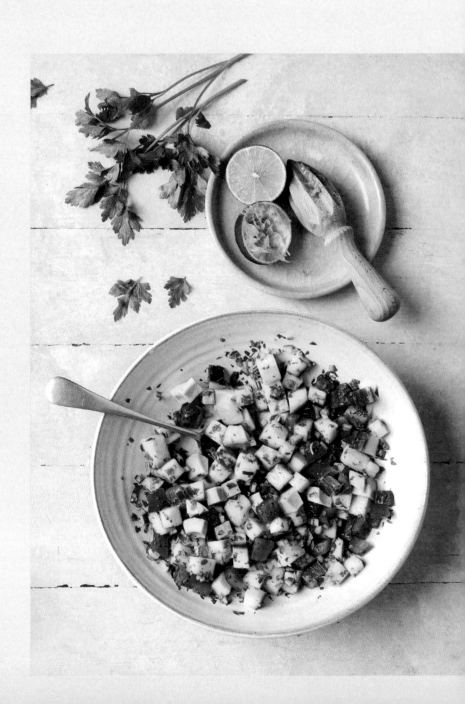

The following sweet and savoury bites offer a delicious selection of ideas for snacks, starters, and sides.

These tasty recipes are easy to assemble or prep in advance, providing inspiration for nutritious and satisfying snacks that will help you feel energized throughout the day on those occasions when energy levels dip between meals. Flex options are also provided in places for vegan and non-vegan choices, or as ideas for adding beneficial nutrients.

Whether you are rustling up a sardine and avocado wrap, for example, or heading out with an easily portable snack such as a slice of banana or broccoli bread, these healthy, low-sugar, home-made light bites will maintain energy levels and stop you reaching for a sugary, processed snack.

As well as being enjoyable stand-alone dishes, recipes such as edamame beans, quinoa tabbouleh, and rainbow salsa also make simple and appetizing starters or sides to complement main meals.

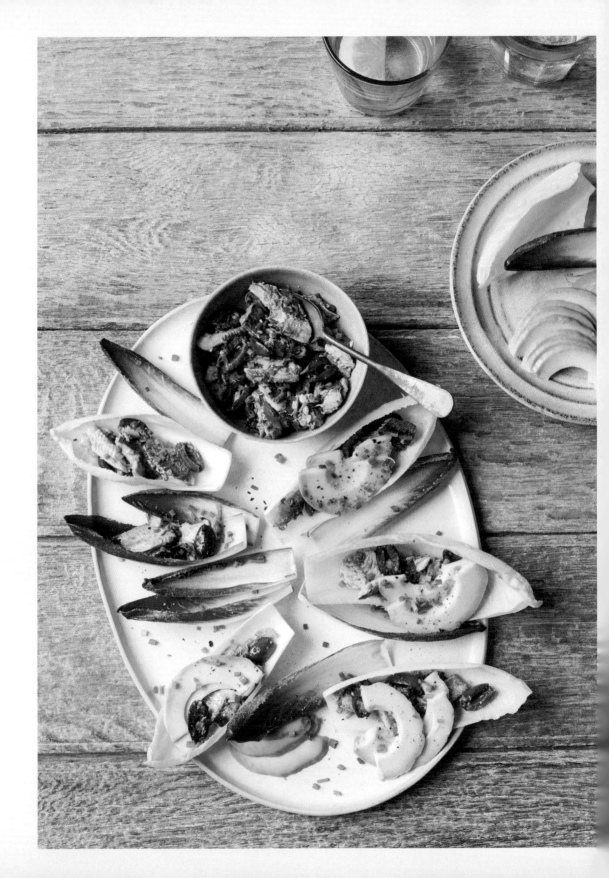

Sardine *and* avocado wrap

supports heart health • provides sustained energy • promotes bone health

Small, flavoursome, and satisfying, sardines are high in heart-protecting omega-3 fatty acids, and the tiny, edible bones are an excellent source of bone-supporting calcium.

Serves 4
Prep 10 mins

240g can whole sardines in olive oil, drained
2 small avocados, pitted and sliced or diced

16 black olives, pitted and halved
juice of 1–2 lemons
20 strands of chives, chopped
1 large head of green chicory, leaves separated

In a bowl, gently break the sardines into chunks, add half the avocado and the remaining ingredients, and toss until well combined. Refrigerate for 1 hour.

Fill each endive leaf with the mixture, dividing it evenly, top with the remaining avocado, and serve.

Tomato *and* garlic toast

supports heart health • helps manage weight • boosts immunity

This traditional Spanish dish has a trio of heart-protecting ingredients with antioxidant-rich tomato, immune-supporting garlic, and the healthy fat source olive oil.

Serves 4
Prep 10 mins

4 slices of bread, ideally gluten-free, about 1.5cm ($\frac{1}{2}$in) thick
2 garlic cloves
2 tomatoes
1–2 tbsp extra virgin olive oil
sea salt and freshly ground black pepper

Toast the bread on both sides until lightly brown and crunchy. Peel the garlic five minutes before using to allow the antibacterial compound allicin to form, maximizing its benefits.

If you have little tolerance for garlic, use the following method. Finely grate the tomatoes into a bowl. Cut the garlic in half and rub it over the toasted bread. Spoon the tomato over the garlicky toast, add a splash of olive oil, and season.

If you digest garlic well, finely grate the tomatoes into a bowl. Crush or grate the garlic and add to the tomatoes. Add the olive oil, season, and mix well. Spoon the tomato mixture over the toasted bread.

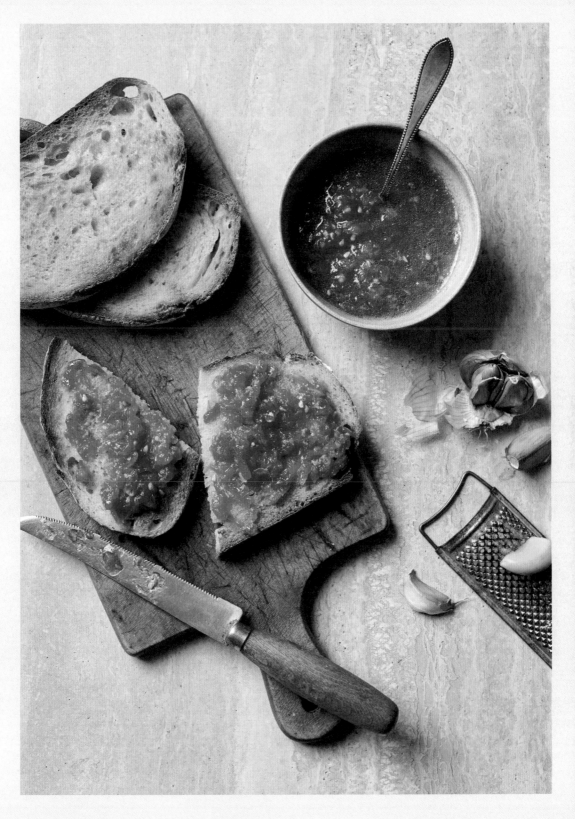

Tomato and garlic toast

Black olive *and* tuna cake

promotes muscle health • helps manage weight • supports digestion

This simple, but filling, snack provides ample muscle-building protein from the tuna, cheese, and eggs, while olives deliver healthy fats as well as fibre to help boost sluggish digestion.

Makes 10 slices
Prep 10 mins
Cook 40 mins

100g (3¹/₂oz) buckwheat flour
1 tsp baking powder
3 eggs

100ml (3¹/₂fl oz) unsweetened milk of your choice
100ml (3¹/₂fl oz) olive oil
100g (3¹/₂oz) black pitted olives, rinsed
100g (3¹/₂oz) Cheddar, grated
2 x 150g can of tuna, drained

Preheat the oven to 180°C (400°F/Gas 6). In a large bowl, add the flour, baking powder, and eggs, then combine using a hand-held electric whisk.

Add the milk and oil and whisk until well combined. Add the olives, Cheddar, and tuna. Combine with a spatula until all the ingredients are well mixed. Pour into a 21 x 11cm (8 x 4in) baking tin. Bake for 40 minutes, or until slightly golden and heated through. Serve warm or enjoy cold.

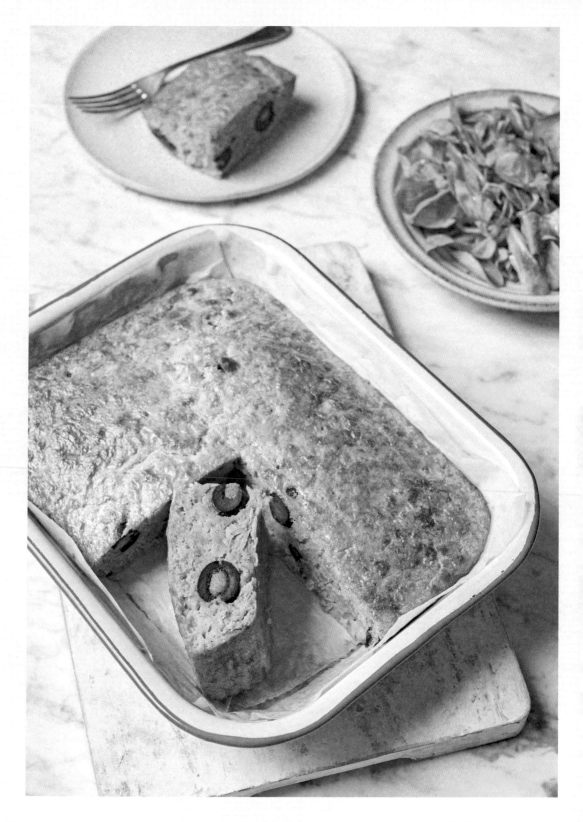

Black olive and tuna cake

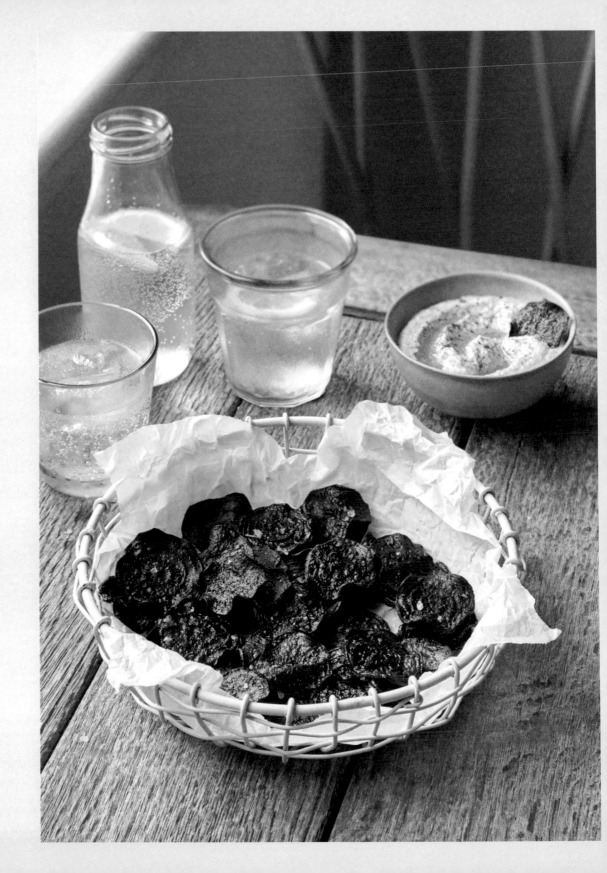

Beetroot crisps

supports heart health • balances hormones • supports metabolism

Vibrant beetroot is high in nitrates, which promote blood vessel and cardio health, and its broad range of antioxidants support liver function, helping to balance hormones and blood sugars.

Serves 4
Prep 10 mins
Cook 15–20 mins
Rest 10 mins

350g (12oz) beetroot, peeled
3 tbsp extra virgin olive oil
1 tsp sea salt
2–3 tbsp rosemary, roughly chopped
hummus, to serve (optional)

Preheat the oven to 190°C (400°C/Gas 6). Use a food processor if available to slice the beetroot consistently, ensuring the slices bake evenly and have the same crisp.

Place the olive oil, salt, and rosemary in a large bowl and combine. Add the beetroot slices and use a brush to spread the oil between them evenly and gently turn them.

Arrange the beetroot slices in a single layer on two baking trays – the slices can touch, but make sure they don't overlap. Bake in the centre of the oven for 15–20 minutes, depending on the thickness of the slices. Watch closely after 10 minutes because they can burn quickly. Leave to cool on a wire rack until crispy before serving. Eat on their own or serve with hummus if desired.

Edamame beans

helps calm hot flushes • promotes muscle health • supports digestion

High in muscle-strengthening protein and fibre, for digestive health, edamame beans are also a key source of phytoestrogens, helping to soothe hot flushes and night sweats.

Serves 4
Prep 5 mins
Cook 3–10 mins

800g (1¾lb) frozen edamame
   with pods, or 400g (14oz)
   without pods
1 tsp extra virgin olive oil
1 garlic clove, crushed
2 tbsp grated Parmesan
sea salt flakes

Cook the edamame according to the packet instructions. Add the olive oil and garlic and toss. Scatter over the Parmesan and sprinkle with salt flakes. Enjoy on their own as a snack or serve as a side.

Quinoa tabbouleh

boosts immunity • has anti-inflammatory properties • balances moods

This gluten-free tabbouleh is high in micronutrients. Quinoa is full of flavonoids, which have anti-inflammatory, anti-viral, cancer-fighting, and mood-balancing properties, promoting overall health in midlife.

Serves 4
Prep 15 mins
Cook 10 mins
Rest 1 hour

60g (2oz) uncooked quinoa
1 small onion, finely diced
100g (3½oz) flat-leaf parsley, leaves separated and stems finely chopped

25g (scant 1oz) mint, leaves separated and stems finely chopped
4 tomatoes, finely diced
40g (1½oz) pomegranate seeds
juice of 2 lemons
1½ tbsp extra virgin olive oil
sea salt and freshly ground black pepper

Cook the quinoa according to the packet instructions. Leave to cool and set aside. Place the onion, parsley, and mint in a serving bowl and add the tomatoes.

Add the quinoa, pomegranate seeds, lemon juice, and olive oil and stir until well combined. Season to taste. Refrigerate for at least 1 hour to let the flavours develop, then serve either on its own or as a side dish.

Broccoli bread

Makes 10 slices
Prep 20 mins
Cook 1 hour
Rest 15 mins

400g (14oz) steamed
    broccoli, blended
70g (2¹/₂oz) ground flaxseeds
40g (1¹/₂oz) chia seeds
30g (1oz) coconut flour
30g (1oz) chickpea
    (gram) flour
3 tbsp coconut oil
¹/₄ tsp freshly ground black
    pepper
¹/₄ tsp sea salt
1 tsp baking powder
120ml (4fl oz) almond milk
10g (¹/₄oz) basil, chopped
30g (1oz) pumpkin seeds

Flex it – *For a non-vegan version,
swap the flaxseeds for 2 eggs.*

helps calm hot flushes • keeps energy levels steady • supports digestion

Cruciferous broccoli has oestrogen-balancing properties and phytoestrogens, to help ease hot flushes. This tasty bread is also full of fibre and healthy fats, keeping blood sugar levels steady.

Preheat the oven to 190°C (400°F/Gas 6). Line a 21 x 11cm (8 x 4in) loaf tin with parchment paper.

Place all the ingredients in a large bowl and combine until they form a dough-like consistency. Place the dough in the loaf tin and bake for 1 hour, or until cooked through and an inserted skewer comes out clean. Leave to cool in the tin before serving. Enjoy warm, or cool completely and toast.

Rainbow salsa

Serves 4
Prep 30 mins
Rest 1 hour

**1 large ripe mango,
  peeled and diced**
1 cucumber, diced
**1 small red onion,
  finely diced**
**1 red pepper, deseeded
  and finely diced**
**1 avocado, pitted
  and diced**
1 large tomato, finely diced
**2 garlic cloves, finely
  chopped**
**25g (scant 1oz) flat-leaf
  parsley or coriander,
  chopped**
$\frac{1}{2}$ tsp sea salt
2 tbsp extra virgin olive oil
juice of 2 limes

**boosts skin health • supports digestion
• supports heart health**

Full of phytonutrients, this colourful side dish also provides plenty of fibre to ease constipation and bloating, while the healthy fats from the avocados and olive oil support skin and heart health.

Place all the ingredients in a large bowl and stir well to combine.

Refrigerate for at least 1 hour to allow the flavours to develop. Enjoy!

(photographed overleaf)

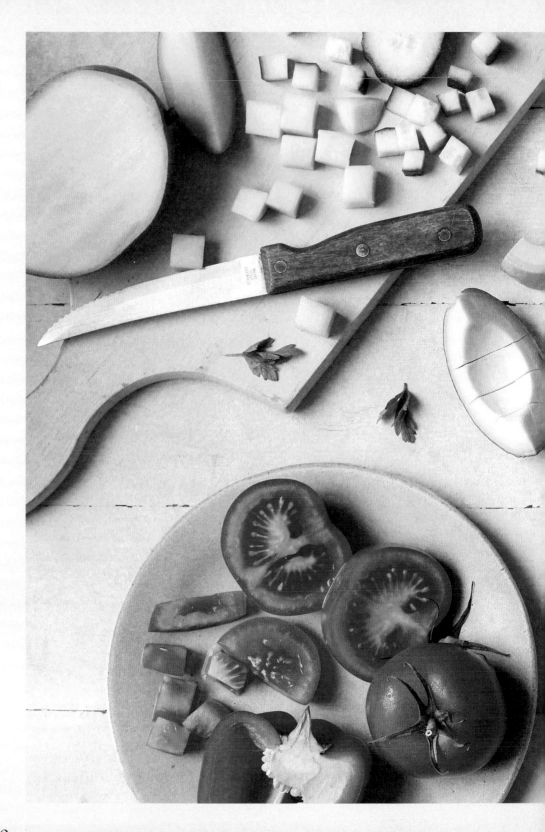

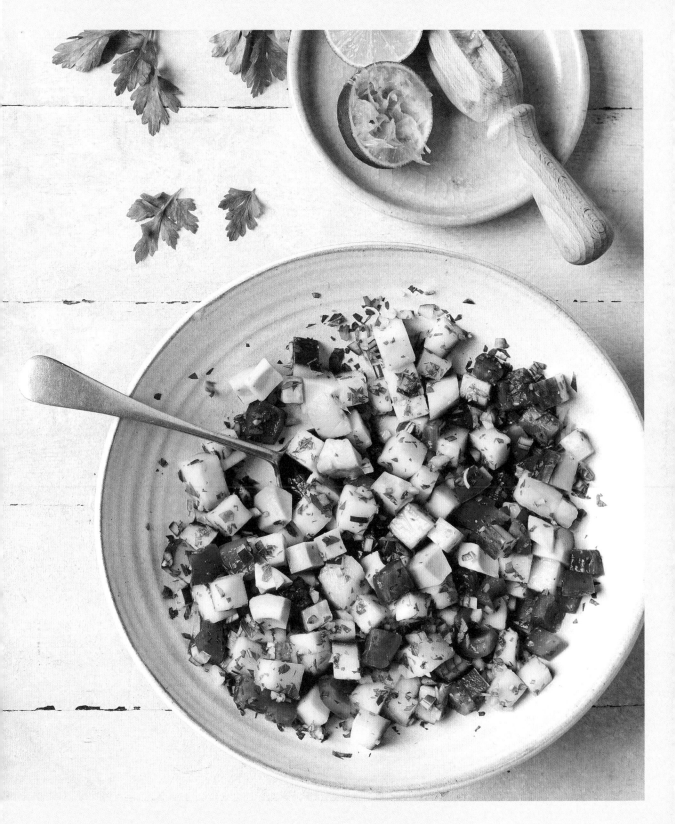

Rainbow salsa

Blueberry *and* apple cookies

Makes about 8
Prep 15 mins
Cook 25–35 mins

1 banana
1 egg
40g (1¹/₂oz) coconut oil,
  melted
1 tbsp maple syrup
100g (3¹/₂oz) buckwheat
  flour
80g (3oz) jumbo oats
1 tsp baking powder
1 tbsp ground flaxseeds
2 apples, cored, peeled,
  and grated
80g (3oz) blueberries

Flex it – *For a vegan version,*
try replacing the egg with
1 tbsp ground flaxseeds and
2¹/₂–3 tbsp water, whisked then
left a few minutes before using.

boosts immunity • provides sustained energy
• supports digestion

Naturally sweet apples and blueberries are full of immune-boosting antioxidants and a good source of soluble fibre, supporting bowel health to help ease menopausal bloating and constipation.

Preheat the oven to 180°C (400°F/Gas 6). Line a baking sheet with parchment paper.

In a large bowl, mash the banana with a fork then add the egg, coconut oil, and maple syrup and whisk well. Add the flour, oats, baking powder, and flaxseeds and stir well. Add the apples and combine well into the mixture. Gently fold in the blueberries.

Use ¹/₃ cup to measure the mixture for each cookie, to ensure they cook evenly. Place the mixture for the cookie on the baking sheet and flatten. Repeat, using up all the dough, to make around 8 cookies in total.

Bake for 25–35 minutes, or until golden. Enjoy the cookies warm or cold.

174

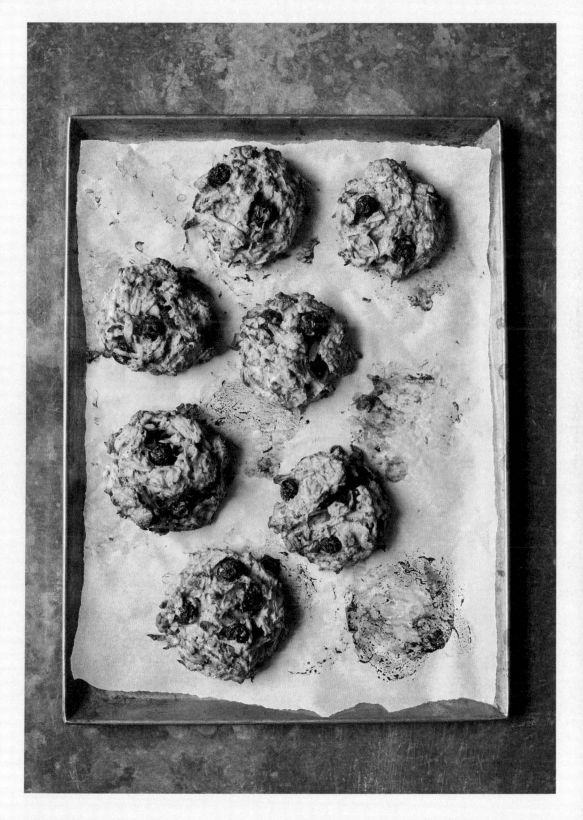

Blueberry and apple cookies

Strawberry coconut muffins

Makes 8
Prep 15 mins
Cook 25 mins
Rest 15 mins

400ml can full-fat
  coconut milk
1 tbsp maple syrup
1 tsp vanilla extract
1 tbsp ground flaxseeds
100g (3¹/₂oz) jumbo oats
20g (³/₄oz) unsweetened,
  shredded coconut
1 tsp baking powder
80g (3oz) strawberries,
  chopped

supports digestion • helps balance hormones • aids cognition

Deliciously moist, these low-sugar muffins have healthy fats to support hormone production and brain health and fibre from the flaxseeds and oats, to regulate bowel movements.

Preheat the oven to 190°C (400°F/Gas 6). Place the coconut milk, maple syrup, vanilla extract, and flaxseeds in a large mixing bowl and mix with a hand-held blender. Leave to rest for 5 minutes.

Add the oats, shredded coconut, and baking powder and combine with a silicon spatula. Carefully fold in the strawberries.

Divide the batter between 8 compartments in a silicon muffin tray and bake for 25 minutes, or until the muffins look bubbly, are golden brown around their edges, and firm to the touch. Leave to cool for 15 minutes before transferring out of the muffin tray. Allow to cool completely then enjoy.

Chocolate chip banana bread

Serves 8
Prep 15 mins
Cook 35 mins
Rest 10 mins

2½ tbsp olive oil
1 large ripe banana, mashed
2 tbsp maple syrup
240ml (8fl oz) unsweetened
 milk of your choice
10g (¼oz) flaxseeds
100g (3½oz) chickpea
 (gram) flour, sieved
15g (½oz) baking powder,
 sieved
40g (1½oz) vegan
 chocolate chips

helps calm hot flushes • supports heart health • helps manage weight

This satisfying snack has phytoestrogens from both the flaxseeds and chickpeas, relieving hot flushes. Bananas promote healthy blood vessels and olive oil adds moisture and supports heart health.

Preheat the oven to 180°C (400°F/Gas 6). Line a 21 x 11cm (8 x 4in) loaf tin with parchment paper. Place the oil, banana, maple syrup, milk, and flaxseeds in a large bowl and stir to combine. Add the flour, baking powder, and half of the chocolate chips, and mix until all the ingredients are well combined.

Pour the mixture into the loaf tin and scatter over the remaining chocolate chips. Bake for 35 minutes, or until an inserted skewer comes out clean. Leave to cool before serving.

Chocolate *and* peanut butter bites

Makes 10
Prep 10 mins
Rest 2 hours

30g (1oz) coconut oil
30g (1oz) maple syrup
10g ($^1/_4$oz) 100 per cent
   cacao powder
45g (1$^1/_2$oz) crunchy
   peanut butter
3 tbsp white sesame
   seeds
3 tbsp unsweetened
   shredded coconut

supports heart health • balances moods • helps manage weight

High in heart-healthy fats and low in sugar, these tasty treats satisfy hunger pangs while keeping blood sugar levels steady.

Place the coconut oil, maple syrup, cacao powder, and peanut butter in a bain-marie and stir until well combined. Cool in the fridge for 1 hour, or until the mixture has hardened.

Prepare two bowls: place the sesame seeds in one bowl and the shredded coconut in the other. Using just under a tablespoon measure, scoop out a small ball from the mixture, then roll it gently over either the sesame seeds or the shredded coconut. Continue to make balls with the rest of the mixture.

Place the balls on a tray and refrigerate for at least 1 hour, or until ready to serve.

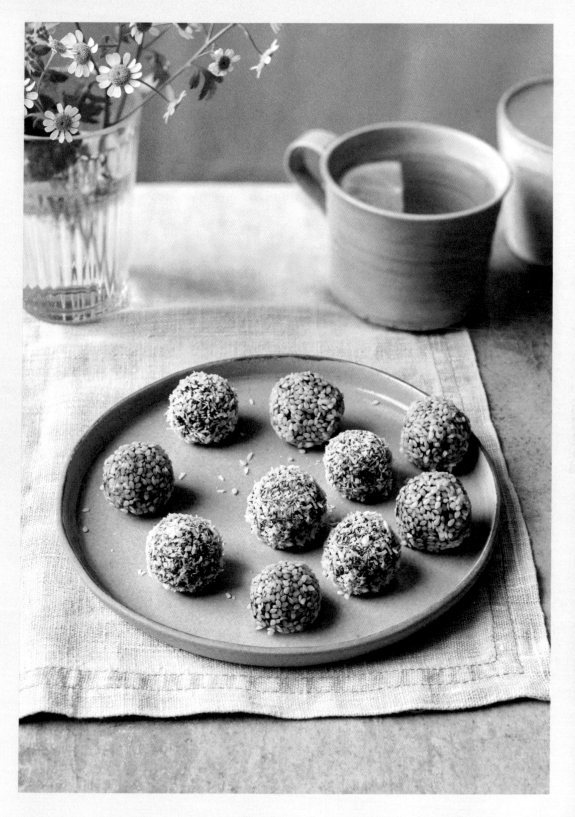

Chocolate and peanut butter bites

Chocolate *and* hazelnut bites

aids cognition • supports heart health • boosts skin health • supports digestion

Cacao in dark chocolate contains powerful antioxidants that have a positive impact on brain, cardiovascular, and digestive health and support cholesterol. Cacao also promotes healthy skin, which can be thinner and drier in the menopause.

Makes 12
Prep 25 mins
Rest 30 mins

50g (1³/₄oz) sliced almonds
50g (1³/₄oz) hazelnuts, roughly chopped

1 tbsp orange juice
zest of 1 orange
100g (3¹/₂oz) dark chocolate, cooking or non-cooking, at least 70 per cent cocoa

Place the almonds, hazelnuts, orange juice, and zest in a bowl and mix together well. Heat a pan over a high heat, add the nut mixture, and heat for a few minutes – tossing regularly to prevent it from burning – until the nuts have darkened slightly. Set aside.

Melt the chocolate in a bain-marie. Add the nut mixture to the melted chocolate and mix well, so that the nuts are covered evenly with the chocolate. Line a plate with parchment paper, make 12 balls (about 15g/¹/₂oz each) from the mixture, and place the balls on the plate. Refrigerate for 30 minutes then enjoy.

Lime *and* blueberry muffins

supports heart health • boosts skin health

These sweet muffins are rich in vitamin E from the almond flour. Vitamin E is excellent for heart and eye health, both of which can deteriorate in midlife, and also helps to nourish skin.

Makes 6
Prep 10 mins
Cook 25 mins
Rest 15 mins

130g (4³/₄oz) almond flour
¹/₂ tsp bicarbonate of soda

pinch of sea salt
zest and juice of 1 lime
2 eggs
1 banana, mashed
2 tbsp maple syrup
100g (3¹/₂oz) blueberries

Preheat the oven to 180°C (400°F/Gas 6). Place the flour, bicarbonate of soda, salt, and lime zest in a bowl and whisk to combine. Stir in the lime juice, eggs, banana, and maple syrup, then fold the blueberries into the mixture.

Divide the batter between 6 compartments in a silicon muffin tray and bake for 25 minutes, or until cooked through and an inserted skewer comes out clean. Remove from the oven and leave to cool in the muffin tray before serving.

Fruit jellies

Serves 4
Prep 10 mins
Cook 5 mins
Rest 30 mins

120ml (4fl oz) bone broth (see p.216)
150g (5¹/₂oz) fruit of choice, fresh or frozen – choose from berries, kiwi, pineapple, mango
1 tbsp lemon juice
12g (¹/₄oz), or 1 sachet, best-quality unflavoured beef gelatine
1–2 tsp honey, to sweeten (optional)

Flex it – *Swap bone broth for water if preferred.*

boosts immunity • boosts skin health • supports healthy bones

These fruity bites are rich in immune-boosting minerals and collagen from the bone broth and gelatine, supporting bone, gut, and skin health.

Place the bone broth, fruit, and lemon juice in a small pan over a medium heat. Bring to the boil, then reduce to a simmer for a couple of minutes until the fruit softens. Turn off the heat and leave to cool for a few minutes, until warm.

Add the gelatine and blend well, adding honey if using, then pour into sweet moulds or small dishes. Alternatively, pour into small ramekins for a jelly-like dessert. Refrigerate for at least 30 minutes.

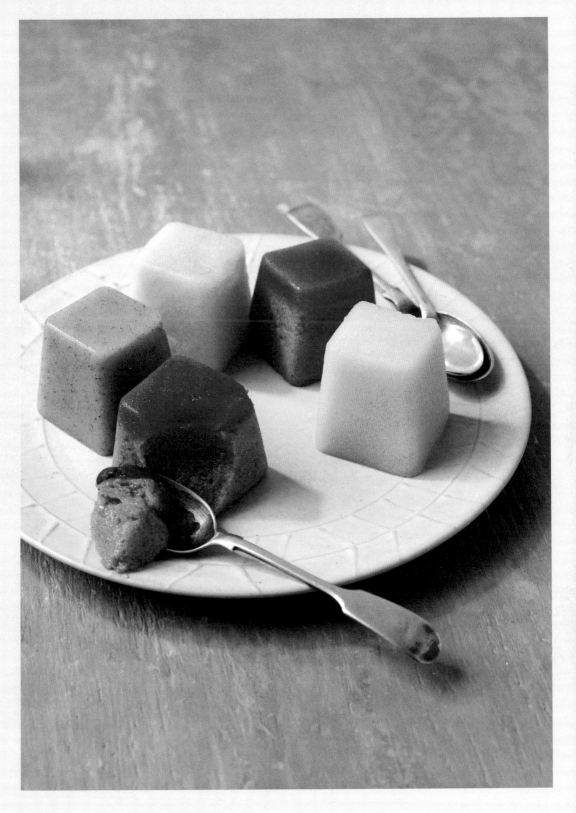

Fruit jellies

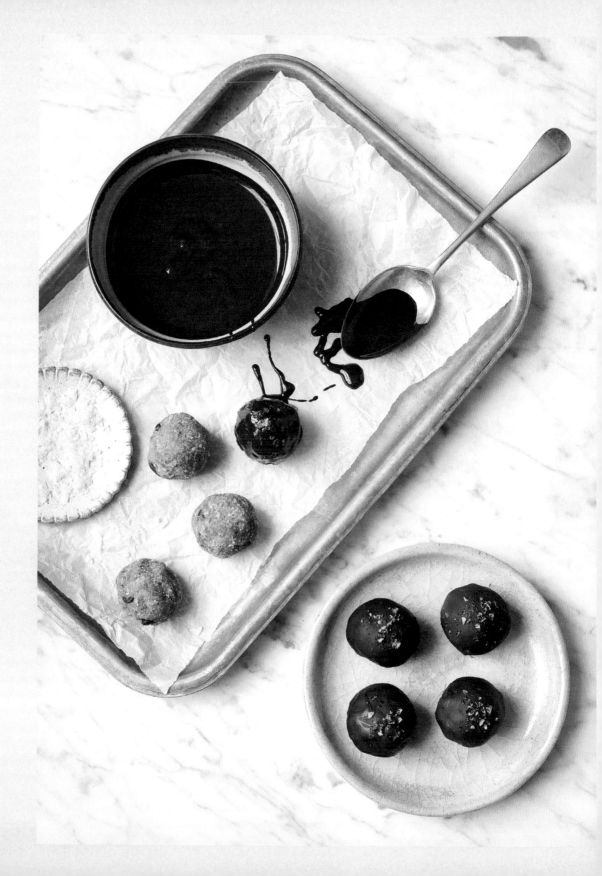

No-bake cookie truffles

Makes 8
Prep 5 mins
Cook 20 mins
Freeze 30 mins

½ tbsp ground flaxseeds
1 tbsp unsweetened milk
   of your choice
30g (1oz) melted coconut oil
30g (1oz) coconut sugar
70g (2½oz) ground almonds
20g (¾oz) coconut flour
¼ tsp sea salt, plus extra to
   sprinkle (optional)
15g (½oz) dark chocolate
   chips
70g (2½oz) dark chocolate,
   at least 70 per cent cocoa

provides sustained energy • helps calm hot flushes • aids cognition

These sweet treats are a healthy way to quash hunger pangs. Flaxseeds provide phytoestrogens, which may ease hot flushes, while anti-inflammatory flavanols in dark chocolate support brain health.

Place the flaxseeds, milk, coconut oil, and coconut sugar in a bowl and combine. Add the ground almonds, coconut flour, and salt, and mix well to form a cookie-dough consistency. Fold in the chocolate chips.

Line a baking sheet with parchment paper. Roll the dough into 8 balls and place these on the baking sheet. Freeze for 10–15 minutes.

In the meantime, slowly melt the chocolate using a bain-marie, stirring frequently to ensure that the chocolate doesn't become lumpy or grainy.

Dip each ball into the melted chocolate, coating them evenly. Place the coated balls on the baking sheet and sprinkle with a little coarse sea salt if desired. Freeze for another 20 minutes before eating. Allow to sit at room temperature for a few minutes then enjoy.

Desserts and bakes

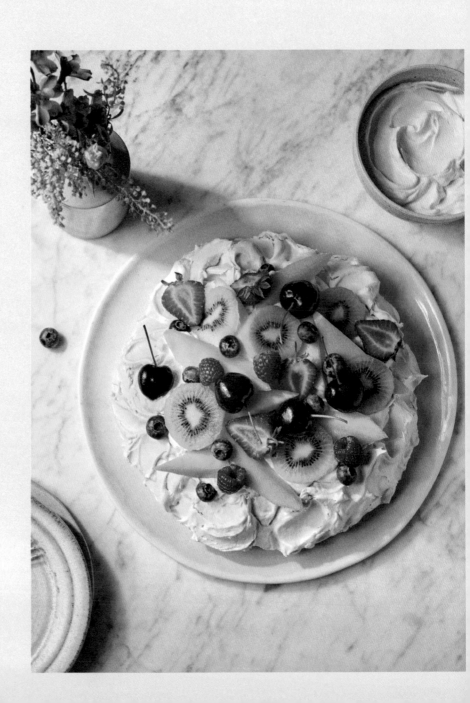

Sweet desserts and bakes may not feature in your diet every day, but they can be an enjoyable part of family meals on occasion and play an important role in celebratory gatherings.

The selection of low-sugar sweet treats in the following section favours natural sweeteners such as fruit and mildly spiced flavouring over highly refined processed sugars. Flex options are also provided in places, offering dairy-free alternatives.

Choose from family favourites such as quick-to-make ice cream, chocolate-dipped fruit platter, fruit-filled crêpes, and blueberry crumble, or opt for simple but delicious desserts such as flaxseed pudding, baked apples, and more. For special occasions, impress the table with a fruit-laden colourful pavlova or bake a succulent cake.

Blueberry crumble

Serves 4
Prep 15 mins
Cook 20–30 mins

300g (10oz) blueberries
juice of 1 lemon
150g (5^1/$_2$oz) ground
  almonds
30g (1oz) macadamia
  nuts, chopped
50g (1^3/$_4$oz) butter, melted
2 tbsp maple syrup
^{1}/$_4$ tsp cinnamon
pinch of sea salt
yogurt, to serve (optional)

supports heart health • aids cognition • boosts immunity

Blueberries have immune-boosting antioxidant flavanols, whose documented anti-inflammatory properties aid heart health and cognition. Crunchy macadamias add healthy fats and protein.

Preheat the oven to 190°C (400°F/Gas 6). Place the blueberries in a 16 x 24cm (6^1/$_2$ x 9^1/$_2$in) baking dish and add half the lemon juice. Toss to combine.

Place all the remaining ingredients, including the remaining lemon juice, in a bowl and stir to combine. Spread the mixture over the blueberries and bake until the blueberries are bubbling and the topping is golden brown, about 20–30 minutes. Add foil if needed to stop the top from burning. Serve warm with a dollop of yogurt if desired.

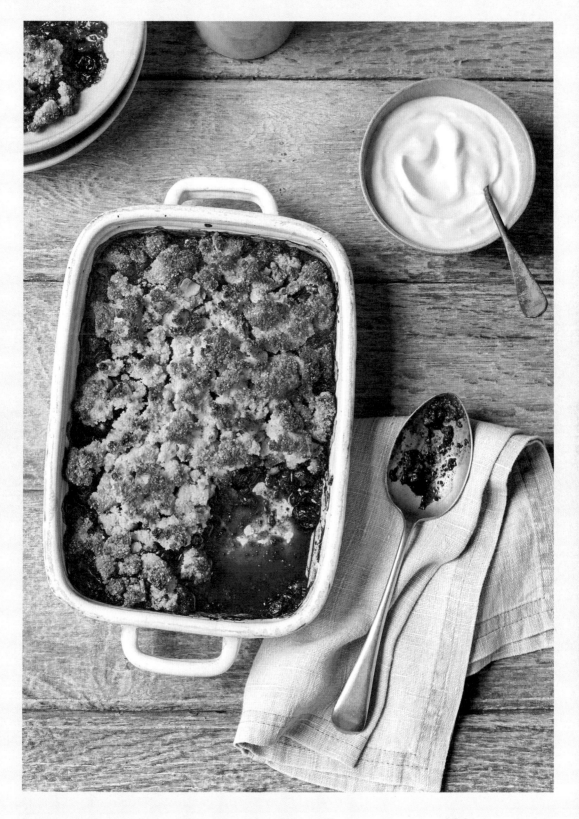

Blueberry crumble

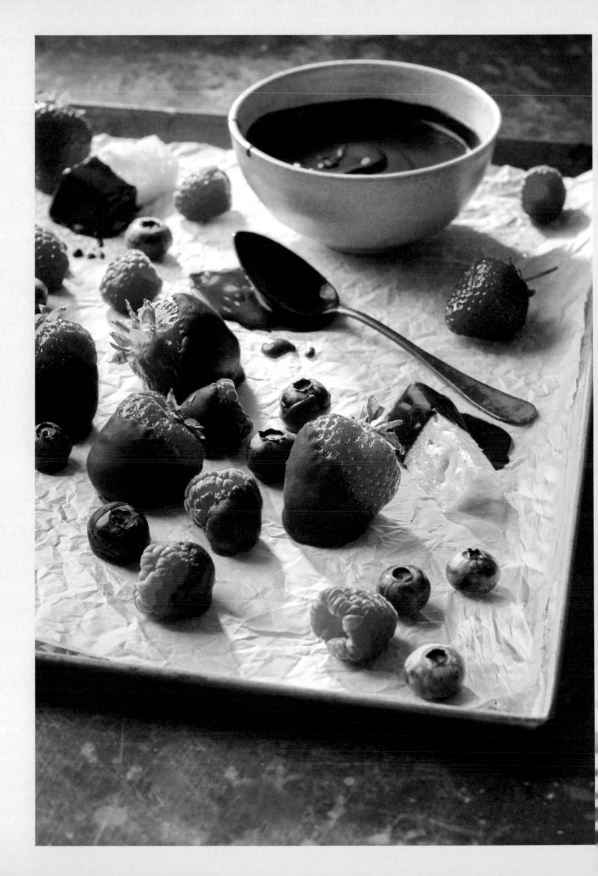

Chocolate-dipped fruit platter

eases constipation • supports heart health • boosts immunity

This delicious combo of dark chocolate and fibrous fruit is an antioxidant-rich treat. Flavanols in dark chocolate and fruit aid immunity and blood vessel health, which can decline in midlife.

Serves 4
Prep 10 mins
Cook 10 mins
Rest 1 hour

400g (14oz) selection of fruits, such as strawberries, banana, apple, pineapple, pear, blueberries, raspberries, clementine
100g (3¹/₂oz) dark chocolate (cooking or non-cooking), at least 70 per cent cocoa
120ml (4fl oz) single cream

Prepare the fruits: strawberries and other summer berries can be used whole; dice harder fruits such as pineapple and apples; slice bananas; and separate clementine segments. If you wish, arrange the fruit on skewers.

Line a dish with parchment paper. In a bain-marie, melt the chocolate and cream. As soon as the chocolate is melted, remove the hot water to prevent the chocolate from turning lumpy or grainy. Stir well.

Use a fork to dip each piece of fruit into the chocolate, then place on the paper. Leave the dish in the fridge for 1 hour for the chocolate to harden. Transfer the chocolate fruits to a serving dish and enjoy.

Flex it – *Swap single cream for a dairy-free one to reduce dairy content if desired.*

Perfect flaxseed pudding

boosts immunity • helps calm hot flushes • supports gut health

Antioxidant-rich berries and probiotic yogurt promote a healthy gut microbiome, supporting overall health and immunity, while lignans in flaxseeds can help ease symptoms such as hot flushes.

Serves 4
Prep 5 mins
Cool 2 hours

120g (4¹/₂oz) ground flaxseeds
2 tbsp ground cinnamon
450ml (15fl oz) unsweetened
   milk of your choice

2 tbsp maple syrup
500g (1lb 2oz) thick plain yogurt,
   unsweetened
150g (5¹/₂oz) raspberries, mashed
150g (5¹/₂oz) raspberries, whole
4 tbsp pecan nuts, chopped

In a small bowl, gently whisk together the flaxseeds, cinnamon, milk, and maple syrup until smooth. Set aside for 10 minutes, then whisk again. Refrigerate for 2 hours.

Using four large transparent glasses, layer one-quarter of the yogurt and one-quarter of the flaxseed mixture in each glass, sandwiching the flaxseed layer between two yogurt layers. Top with the mashed raspberries and a few whole raspberries, then sprinkle over the pecans.

Flex it – *Opt for plant milk and non-dairy yogurt for a vegan pudding.*

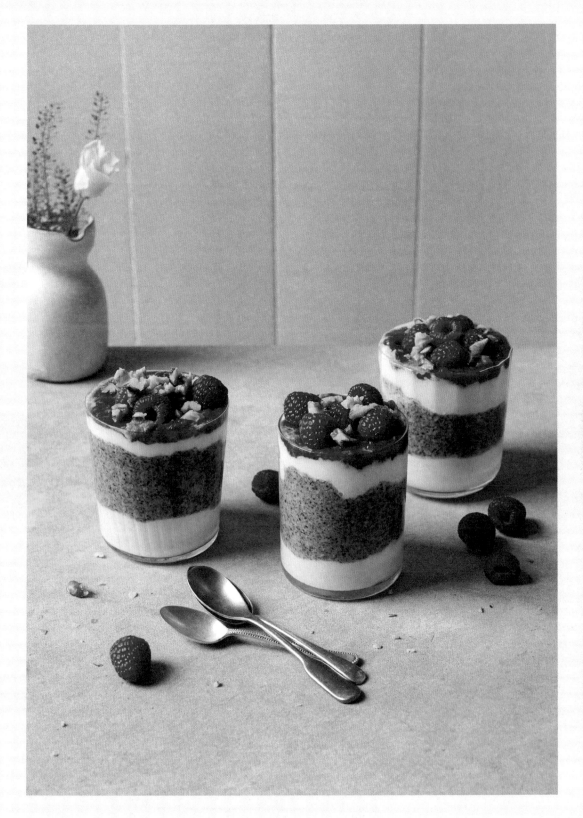

Perfect flaxseed pudding

Baked crème pâtissière

Serves 4
Prep 5 mins
Cook 45 mins
Rest 5 mins

4 eggs
1 tsp vanilla extract
50g (1³/₄oz) sugar
600ml (1 pint) whole milk,
   warm
¹/₄ tsp grated nutmeg
fresh berries, to serve

balances moods • supports muscle health
• promotes bone health

Silky in texture, this high-protein dessert aids muscle and bone health. With sweetness provided by the berries and nutmeg and minimal sugar, it also avoids energy dips to keep moods balanced.

Preheat the oven to 160°C (350°F/Gas 4). Place the eggs, vanilla, and sugar in a large bowl and whisk with a hand-held blender, then slowly add the warm milk. Pour the mixture into a 23cm (9in) round cake tin and sprinkle with the nutmeg.

Bake in the oven in a bain-marie: place the cake tin inside a baking tray, add boiling water to the tray, and bake for 45 minutes in the centre of the oven. Remove from the oven and rest for 5 minutes before serving. Serve with fresh berries, such as blackberries.

Pavlova

Serves 4
Prep 15 mins
Cook 1 hour
Cool 20 mins

For the meringue
1 tsp apple cider vinegar
$^1/_2$ tsp cornflour
2 egg whites
80g (3oz) caster sugar

For the topping
150ml (5fl oz) double cream
300g (10oz) fruits of your
choice, chopped, sliced,
or whole

Flex it – *Use dairy-free cream if preferred.*

promotes gut health • aids digestion

Prebiotic apple cider vinegar feeds good gut bacteria, while antioxidant-rich fruit supplies fibre, easing symptoms such as constipation.

Preheat the oven to 180°C fan (400°F/Gas 6). Line a baking sheet with parchment paper and draw a 20cm (8in) diameter circle on it. Place the apple cider vinegar and cornflour in a bowl and stir well. Place the egg whites in a large bowl and whisk with an electric hand mixer for 5 minutes, or until they form stiff peaks. Add the sugar a tablespoon at a time and whisk for 1 minute after each addition.

Add the apple cider vinegar mix to the egg whites and stir carefully with a spatula. Gently transfer the mixture to the baking sheet. Shape it into the circle, ensuring that the edges are taller and there is a dip in the centre.

Place the pavlova in the oven, reduce the heat to 100°C fan (250°F/Gas $^1/_2$), and bake for 1 hour, or until dry. Turn off the heat and leave in the oven to cool. Once cool, add the topping. Whisk the cream for 1–2 minutes, until you have the desired texture. Spoon into the centre of the pavlova and arrange the fruits on top.

(photographed overleaf)

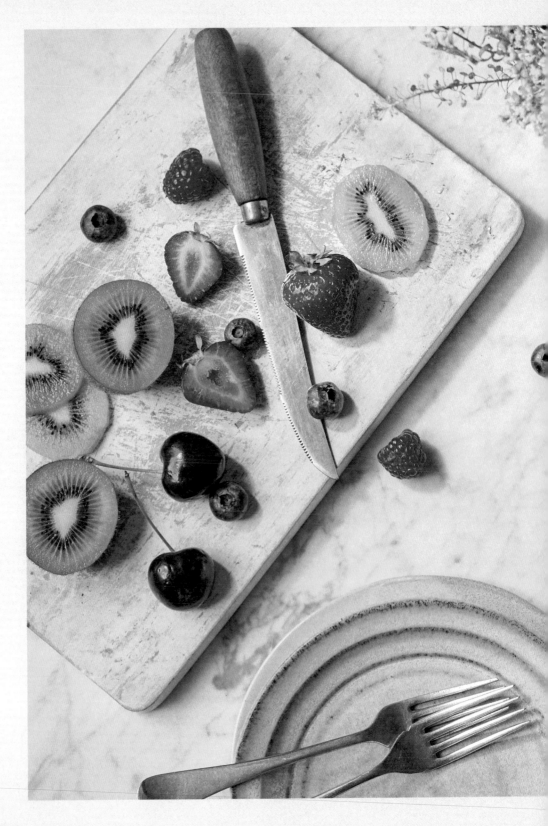

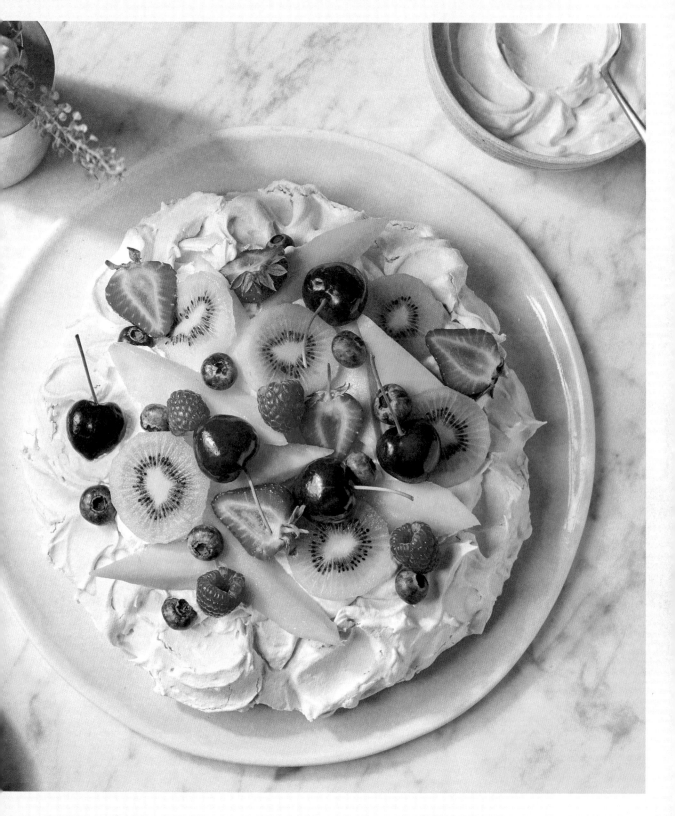

Pavlova

Orange cake

boosts immunity • supports digestion • boosts skin health

Flavourful and moist, this irresistible orange cake provides antioxidant vitamin C to support immunity and collagen production. Fibre-rich almonds supply heart-healthy omega-6 fats, proteins, and skin-supporting vitamin E.

Serves 4
Prep 15 mins
Cook 2 hours
Rest 1 hour

1 small orange, about 200g (7oz)
3 eggs
100ml (3¹/₂fl oz) honey
100g (3¹/₂oz) ground almonds
¹/₂ tsp salt
¹/₂ tsp bicarbonate of soda

Boil the unpeeled orange for 1–1½ hours, or until soft. Quarter the orange and blend it (including the peel) in a food processor until it is smooth.

Preheat the oven to 190°C (400°F/Gas 6) and line a 23cm (9in) round cake tin with parchment paper.

Place all the remaining ingredients, including the blended orange, in a large bowl and whisk together until well combined, then pour the batter into the pan. Bake for 35 minutes, or until an inserted skewer comes out clean. Cool in the pan for 1 hour before serving.

Yogurt cake

aids sleep • supports muscle health • promotes bone health

This simple cake provides a protein boost from the yogurt, supporting muscles and bones, as well as probiotics for a healthy gut. Dairy is also high in tryptophan, the precursor to the sleep-promoting compounds serotonin and melatonin.

Serves 4
Prep 10 mins
Cook 40 mins
Rest 10 mins

150g (5½oz) plain, unsweetened
   live yogurt
60g (2oz) extra virgin olive oil
150g (5½oz) sugar
200g (7oz) self-raising
   gluten-free flour
3 eggs

Preheat the oven to 180°C (400°F/Gas 6). Line a 23cm (9in) round cake tin with parchment paper. Place the yogurt in a bowl then gently mix in the oil, followed by the sugar, flour, and then the eggs, mixing in each ingredient as it is added before adding the next ingredient.

Pour the mixture into the cake tin and bake for 40 minutes, or until an inserted skewer comes out clean. Leave to cool before serving.

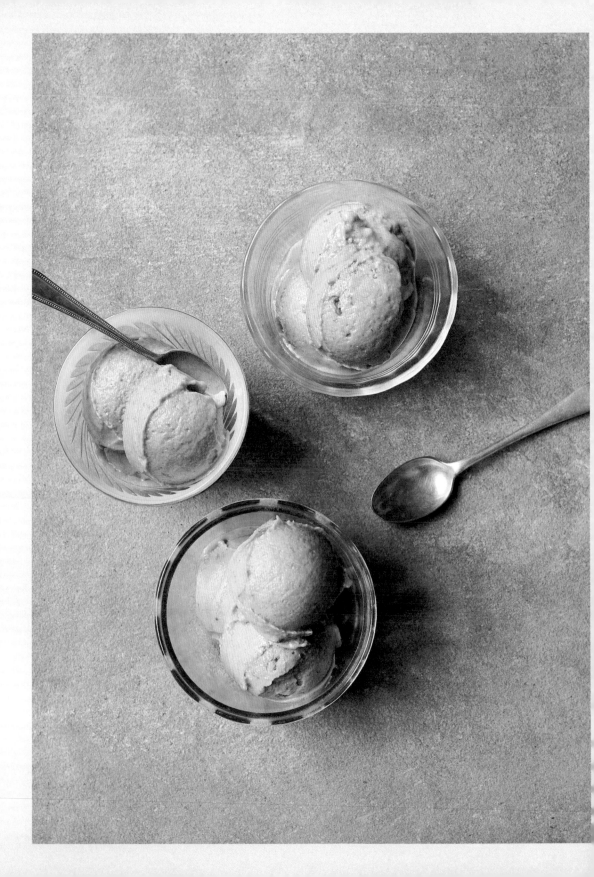

Raspberry ice cream

helps calm hot flushes • boosts immunity • promotes healthy joints

This refreshing ice cream can be soothing for hot flushes. Raspberries are high in antioxidants, aiding immunity, and also contain anti-inflammatory anthocyanins to support joint health during the menopause.

Serves 4
Prep 10 mins
Freeze 4 hours

2 bananas
150g (5¹/₂oz) frozen raspberries

25g (scant 1oz) peanut butter
120ml (4fl oz) unsweetened milk of your choice
¹/₂–1 tbsp clear honey or maple syrup, to sweeten (optional)

Peel the bananas, cut them into 4 portions, and place them in a bag in the freezer for 4 hours (or overnight), until frozen.

Place the bananas, raspberries, peanut butter, and 60ml (2fl oz) of the milk in a food processor and blend.

Add the remaining milk and blend until smooth. Add more milk if needed to achieve the desired texture. Scoop into serving bowls, adding honey or maple syrup to sweeten, if desired.

Simply baked apples

Serves 4
Prep 10 mins
Cook 20–40 mins

40g (1¹/₂oz) butter or ghee, melted
2 tbsp nuts of your choice, roughly chopped
2 tbsp sultanas or dried cranberries
a pinch of cinnamon
4 large apples, ideally Bramley or Granny Smith, cored
yogurt, to serve (optional)

supports metabolism • promotes gut health • balances moods

The humble apple is a good source of soluble fibre to support bowel function. In addition, its natural sugars help stabilize blood sugar levels, helping reduce the risk of diabetes in menopause.

Preheat the oven to 190°C (400°F/Gas 6). In a bowl, mix together the butter, nuts, sultanas, and cinnamon.

Stand up the apples side by side in a baking dish, ensuring that they stay upright. With a spoon or your fingers, stuff each apple with the mixture. Use a spoon or brush to scrape butter left on the sides of the bowl and dab the butter onto the apples.

Bake for 20–40 minutes, until the apples are cooked through, tender, and slightly caramelized. The cooking time will vary depending on the apple variety. Serve the apples warm, on their own or with a dollop of yogurt.

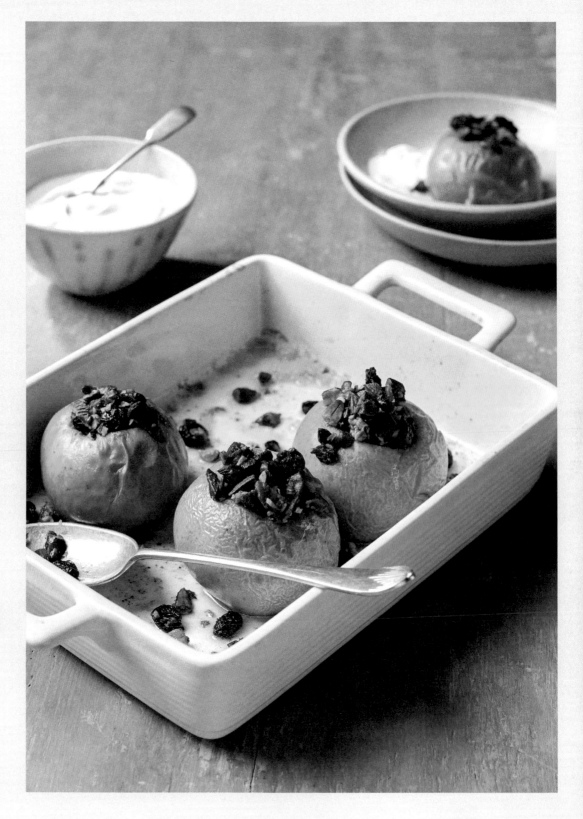

Simply baked apples

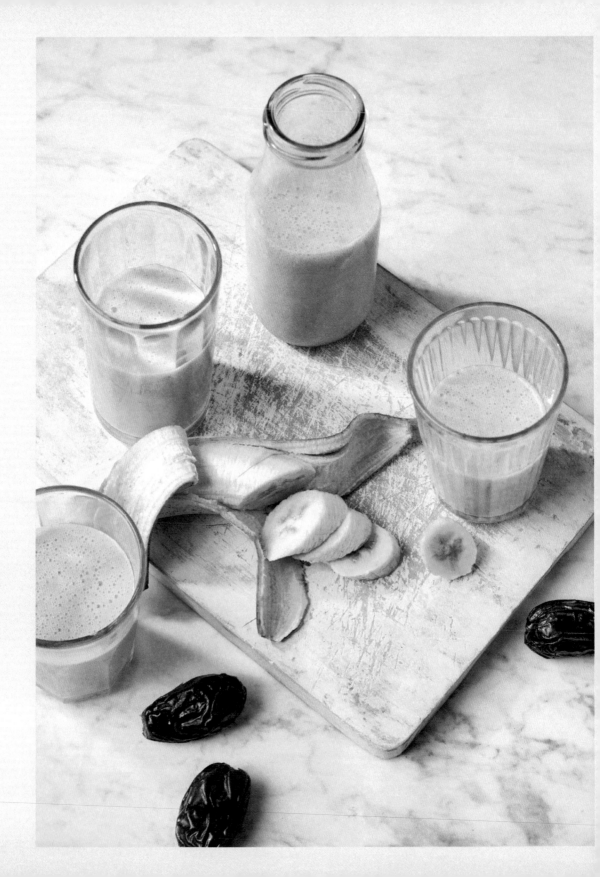

Chai milkshake

boosts immunity • supports digestion • promotes gut health

The blend of warm spices in chai – cinnamon, ginger, nutmeg, cardamom, cloves, star anise, pepper, and coriander – provide immune-boosting antioxidants, while bananas and dates add natural sweetness as well as prebiotics and fibre for gut health.

Serves 4
Prep 5 mins

4 tsp chai mix
6 bananas, peeled, chopped, and frozen
1 litre (1³/₄ pints) unsweetened almond milk, or unsweetened milk of your choice
4 dates, pitted

Place all the ingredients in a blender and blitz until smooth. Taste and add more chai spice mix if desired, or add an extra date to sweeten if necessary.

Chocolate and chia pudding

Serves 4
Prep 15 mins
Rest 20 mins

80g (3oz) chia seeds
240ml (8fl oz)
   unsweetened milk
   of your choice
2 tbsp 100 per cent cocoa
   powder
320g (11oz) unsweetened
   coconut yogurt
4 large strawberries, or
   fruit of your choice

Flex it – *Use a thick, creamy dairy yogurt to up the dairy content here.*

supports heart health • aids cognition • helps calm hot flushes • promotes healthy joints

This light pudding supplies essential omega-3s from the chia seeds, supporting heart and brain health and easing problems such as joint pain. Chia also has phytoestrogens to help combat hot flushes.

Place the chia seeds, milk, and cocoa powder in a large bowl and whisk gently until all the ingredients are well combined. Refrigerate for 20 minutes, or until the chia seeds have absorbed the milk and the mixture is thicker.

Use 4 transparent glasses. For each glass, start with a layer of chia seeds, followed by a layer of yogurt, and repeat. Finish by slicing a strawberry, or fruit of your choice, on top. Enjoy!

Sweet crêpes

butter or ghee (optional)

For the crêpes
100g (3¹/₂oz) buckwheat or other gluten-free flour
400ml (14fl oz) unsweetened milk of your choice
2 eggs

Suggestions for fillings (per crêpe)
strawberries and crème fraîche
lemon juice
pear or strawberry and melted chocolate, with sliced almonds
ricotta and mango
apple and cinnamon

helps manage weight • supports digestion • boosts immunity

These delicious crêpes satisfy the appetite. They are also full of immune-boosting antioxidants from the buckwheat and fruit, supply fibre, and have plenty of muscle-building protein.

For the crêpes, place the flour, milk, and eggs in a food processor and blend until smooth.

Heat a 23cm (9in) frying pan over a medium heat. If you wish, add a knob of butter or ghee, then tilt the pan in a circular motion so the butter coats the pan evenly. This stops the first crêpe sticking to the pan and adds colour and flavour.

Slowly add a ladle, about 100ml (3¹/₂fl oz), of the mixture to the pan and tilt the pan to swirl the mixture and make sure it coats the surface evenly.

Cook each crêpe for about 2 minutes, until the batter bubbles and the bottom is light brown. Loosen with a spatula, turn, and cook the other side for 1–2 minutes. Plate and add the topping of choice to serve.

Banana, raspberry, *and* chocolate ice cream

Serves 1 per flavour option
Prep 5 mins
Freeze 4 hours

Banana flavour
2 bananas
4 tbsp unsweetened milk
   of your choice
¹/₂ tsp vanilla extract
   (optional)
honey or maple syrup,
   to sweeten (optional)

Raspberry flavour
1 banana
120g (4oz) frozen raspberries
4 tbsp unsweetened milk of
   your choice
honey or maple syrup,
   to sweeten (optional)

Chocolate flavour
1 banana
4 tbsp unsweetened milk
   of your choice
1¹/₂ tbsp 100 per cent raw
   unsweetened cacao powder
1 tbsp clear honey or maple
   syrup

helps calm hot flushes • aids cognition • boosts immunity • supports heart health

Naturally cooling and refreshing, this hydrating ice cream is helpful for taking the heat out of hot flushes. The fruits provide fibre and antioxidants for immunity, cognition, and heart health.

Peel the bananas, cut them into 4 portions, and place them in a bag in the freezer for 4 hours (or overnight), until the banana is frozen.

For each flavour, blend or pulse all the ingredients together in a food processor until smooth. If necessary, scrape the sides of the blender and pulse again. Add extra milk to obtain the desired consistency and honey or maple syrup to sweeten, if desired. Scoop into a bowl and enjoy straight away.

Cinnamon apple tart

Serves 4
Prep 25 mins
Cook 45–60 mins

For the pastry
150g (5¹/₂oz) walnuts
1 large egg
10g (¹/₄oz) coconut flour
¹/₄ tsp sea salt

For the filling
700g (1lb 10oz) apples,
    peeled, cored, and sliced
    in 3mm (¹/₈in) slices
1 tbsp lemon juice
1 tbsp cornflour
1 tbsp clear honey
1 tbsp cinnamon

keeps energy levels steady • boosts immunity • supports digestion

Juicy, naturally sweet, and full of flavour, this tart provides immune-supporting vitamin C and fibre from the apples, and heart-healthy omega-3s from the walnuts.

Preheat the oven to 190°C (400°F/Gas 6). To make the pastry crust, pulse the walnuts in a food processor until they are the texture of coarse gravel. Place the walnut mix and the remaining pastry ingredients in a large bowl and mix well to form a ball. Line a 23cm (9in) tart tin with parchment paper. Using wet fingers, press the pastry into the bottom and around the sides of the tin.

Place all the filling ingredients in a large bowl and toss to combine. Fan the apples out on top of the pastry, forming a small circle at the centre and a wider circle around it. Bake for 45–60 minutes, until the apples are cooked and the pastry is golden brown. Serve warm or cold.

Fruit clafoutis

balances moods • supports digestion • helps manage weight

With just a small amount of sugar, the sweetness here comes from the fruits, keeping blood sugar levels steady and also providing antioxidants and digestion-supporting fibre.

Serves 4
Prep 5 mins
Cook 40–45 mins

300g (10oz) fruits, frozen or fresh
4 eggs

100g (3¹/₂oz) gluten-free flour
250ml (9fl oz) whole milk, or unsweetened milk of your choice
50–75g (1³/₄–2¹/₂oz) sugar
yogurt, to serve (optional)

Preheat the oven to 190°C (400°F/Gas 6). Line a 23cm (9in) round oven tin with parchment paper. Place the fruits evenly in the oven tin.

In a bowl, whisk together the eggs, flour, milk, and sugar until smooth, then pour the mixture over the fruits. Bake for 40–45 minutes, until cooked through and golden on top. Serve warm or cold, with a dollop of yogurt if desired.

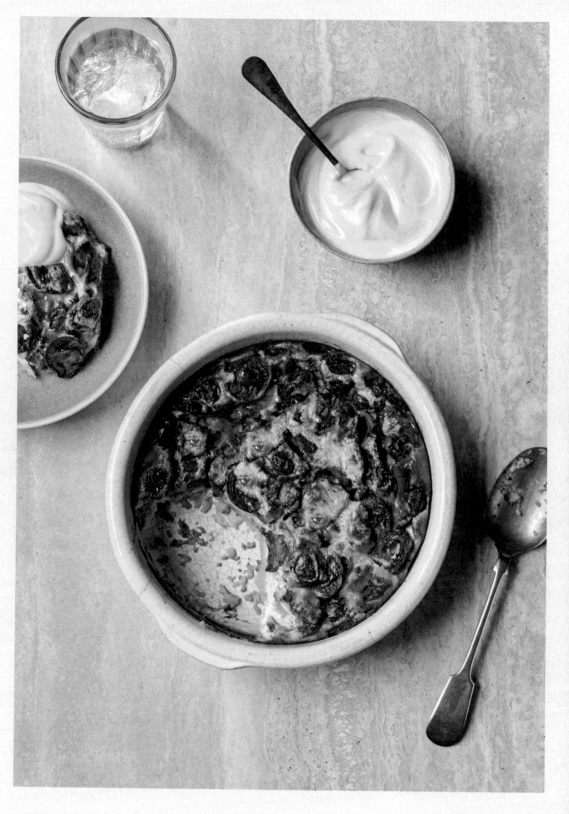

Fruit clafoutis

Drinks

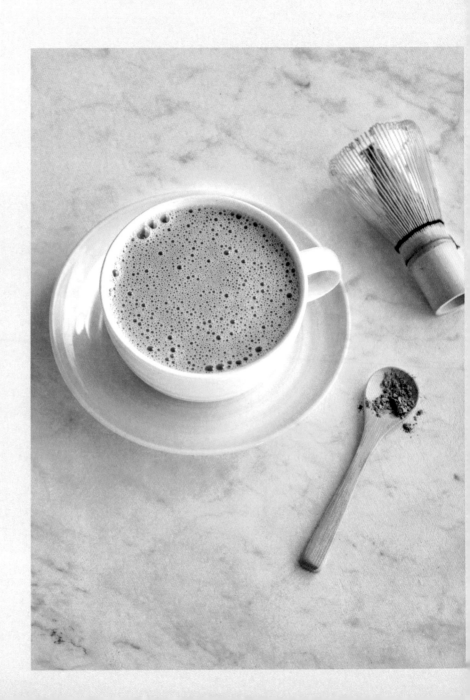

Water is the most important and effective fluid for keeping you well hydrated throughout the day, but at times you may prefer a hot drink or some added flavour.

This selection of hot and cold drinks offers flavourful and soothing alternatives to coffee and tea, but without the diuretic effects and the caffeine spike of coffee.

Mildly spiced, sweet golden milk is a delicious and calming hot beverage, while matcha green tea provides a gentle dose of caffeine, providing calm, lasting energy rather than the quick caffeine hit and subsequent energy dip of coffee. Mineral-rich bone broth and probiotic tangy kombucha provide rich and complex flavours in addition to their impressive nutritional benefits. These healthy and satisfying drinks are the perfect companion to a nourishing and sustaining diet.

Golden milk

Serves 4
Prep 2 mins
Cook 5 mins

1 litre (1³/₄ pints)
unsweetened milk
of your choice
1¹/₄ tbsp ground turmeric
2 tsp ground ginger
2 tsp cinnamon
1¹/₄ tbsp clear honey

Flex it – *To intensify the flavour, replace ground turmeric and ginger with finely grated turmeric and ginger root. A ¹/₄–1 tsp of ground spice is equivalent to 1 tbsp freshly grated root. The flavours are much stronger, so start with a little then build up. To improve gut health, swap milk for bone broth (see p.216).*

helps calm hot flushes • balances moods
• eases nausea

This soothing drink is a great coffee alternative. With anti-inflammatory properties, turmeric, ginger, and cinnamon promote heart and brain health and ease symptoms such as joint pain.

Place all the ingredients in a food processor and blend until well combined.

Pour into a small pan and heat for 3–5 minutes over a medium heat, until hot but not boiling. Serve immediately.

Green tea latte

Serves 4
Prep 2 mins
Cook 5 mins

**1 litre (1³/₄ pints)
unsweetened milk
of your choice**
**4g (¹/₈oz) matcha green
tea powder, or
4 individual sachets**
1 tbsp clear honey
20g (³/₄oz) coconut oil

Flex it – *If you wish, add
10g (¹/₄oz) unflavoured collagen
powder, or 1 individual sachet
collagen per person to up
the collagen content to support
skin, hair, and nail health.*

**eases anxiety • enhances concentration
• balances moods • energizes**

Energizing, antioxidant-high matcha has all the benefits of coffee without the side effects. Adding coconut oil provides nourishing fats and boosts collagen production for healthy skin and nails.

Place the milk and green tea powder in a food processor and blend until well combined.

Transfer to a small pan and heat for 3–5 minutes over a medium heat, until hot but not boiling. Add the honey and coconut oil, stir, and serve immediately or leave to cool as preferred.

Bone broth

Makes 2–3 litres (3¹/₂–5¹/₄ pints)
Prep 5 mins
Cook 3–12 hours

**bones, carcass, skin, and
knuckles of 1 whole
roasted chicken (all the
non-flesh parts that
have not been eaten)**
**2 tbsp raw apple cider
vinegar**
**sea salt and freshly
ground black pepper**

Flex it – *Add onion, garlic,
and other root vegetables for
extra nutrients.*

**promotes bone health • boosts immunity
• supports digestion • promotes healthy joints**

A base to many recipes, this can also be enjoyed as
a warming substitute for coffee. With cholesterol,
collagen, and minerals, this supports immunity,
joints, and bone health, and promotes a healthy gut.

Place all the ingredients in a large pan and add 4 litres
(7 pints) of water. Bring to the boil, then reduce to
a simmer and cover. Cook for at least 3–5 hours, and
up to 12 hours, or until reduced by around a half. The
flavours will intensify the more the broth is reduced.

Strain and discard the bones. Either use immediately
or store in glass jars in the fridge for up to 1 week.
Alternatively, freeze for 1–2 months in a plastic bottle,
leaving 5cm (2in) at the top of the jar to allow for
expansion in the freezer.

Kombucha

Makes 3 litres (5¹/₄ pints)
Prep 10 mins
Rest 7 days

200g (7oz) granulated sugar
8 bags of black tea, green
tea, or a mix (or 2
tablespoons of loose tea)
1 scoby per fermentation jar

boosts immunity • supports digestion
• aids cognition • eases anxiety

This fermented drink is a fantastic source of probiotics, supplying healthy gut bacteria. Optimizing gut health aids nutrient absorption, immunity, and cognition and promotes wellbeing.

In a large bowl, dissolve the sugar in 3 litres (5¹/₄ pints) of hot, boiled water. Add the tea. Once the tea is cool, remove the tea bags or strain the loose tea.

Pour the mixture into a sterilized large glass jar and gently place the scoby inside. Cover the top of the jar with a muslin cloth or paper towel and secure with a rubber band.

Store the jar in a cupboard. After seven days, start to test the kombucha flavour daily by pouring a little into a cup. Once you are happy with the balance of sweetness and tartness, remove the scoby, transfer the kombucha to a bottle, and refrigerate, ready to drink.

Index

Resources

10–11 The menopause years
Menopause: diagnosis and
management
https://www.nice.org.uk/guidance/ng23/
https://www.daisynetwork.org/
about-poi/what-is-poi/

12–13 Your hormones now
Menopause and diabetes
https://www.diabetes.co.uk/
menopause-and-diabetes.html
Infographic, p13
https://nutritionalbalancing.org/
center/htma/conditions/articles/
menopause
https://my.clevelandclinic.org/health/
diseases/15224-menopause-
perimenopause-and-postmenopause
https://www.health.harvard.edu/

womens-health/perimenopause--
rocky-road-to-menopause
https://proovtest.com/blogs/blog/do-
progesterone-levels-decrease-with-age

14–17 Menopausal symptoms
Menopause, perimenopause, and
postmenopause
https://my.clevelandclinic.org/health/
diseases/15224-menopause-
perimenopause-and-postmenopause
What factors influence how long
menopause lasts?
https://www.verywellhealth.com/
how-long-will-menopause-
last-2322698

20–21 Reviewing your diet
Hurrell R, Egli I, "Iron bioavailability
and dietary reference values", *The*

American Journal of Clinical Nutrition,
2010, 91 (5), 1461S–1467S
https://academic.oup.com/ajcn/
article/91/5/1461S/4597424
Biondi B, Klein I, "Hypothyroidism as
a risk factor for cardiovascular
disease", *Endocrine*. 2004, 24 (1), 1–13
https://pubmed.ncbi.nlm.nih.
gov/15249698/
Osteoporosis and menopause
https://www.webmd.com/menopause/
guide/osteoporosis-menopause
Massier V et al, "Menopause and
sarcopenia: a potential role for sex
hormones", *Maturitas*. 2011, 68 (4),
331–6
Bioavailability
https://www.merriam-webster.com/
dictionary/bioavailability

22–3 Staying nourished in the menopause
Stachenfeld NS, "Hormonal changes during menopause and the impact on fluid regulation", *Reproductive Science*. 2014, 21 (5), 555–61 *https://pubmed.ncbi.nlm.nih.gov/24492487/*
Prevent disease and fight aging with micronutrients
https://draxe.com/nutrition/micronutrients/
Genetic factors impacting nutritional requirement
https://www.news-medical.net/health/Genetic-Factors-Impacting-Nutritional-Requirement.aspx

24–27 Eat more protein
Should you boost your protein intake as you age?
https://aaptiv.com/magazine/protein-intake-age
Santarpia L et al, "Dietary protein content for an optimal diet: a clinical view", *Journal of Cachexia, Sarcopenia and Muscle*. 2017, 8 (3), 345–348
https://www.ncbi.nlm.nih.gov/pmc/articles/PMC5476844/
Amino acids
https://www.medicinenet.com/10_foods_high_in_essential_amino_acids/article.htm

28–31 Choose the right fats
Lipids
https://pressbooks-dev.oer.hawaii.edu/humannutrition/chapter/the-functions-of-lipids-in-the-body/
Cholesterol
https://www.heartuk.org.uk/cholesterol/what-is-cholesterol
Steroid pathways
https://dutchtest.com/wp-content/uploads/2017/10/Steroid-Pathways.pdf
Infographic, p31
https://www.ars.usda.gov/ARSUserFiles/80400535/Data/SR/SR28/reports/sr28fg04.pdf

32–35 Rethink carbohydrates
Infographic, p33
https://www.health.harvard.edu/diseases-and-conditions/glycemic-index-and-glycemic-load-for-100-foods
https://documents.hants.gov.uk/hms/

HealthyEatingontheRun-LowGlycemicIndexFoodList.pdf
https://linaleaner.health.blog/2017/07/06/g-i-glycemic-index/
https://nutritiondata.self.com/topics/glycemic-index

36–39 Increase your vegetable and fruit intake
Lindre MC et al, "Iron and copper homeostasis", *Biometals*, 2003. 16: 145–160
https://link.springer.com/article/10.1023/A:1020729831696
Beetroot *https://www.todaysdietitian.com/newarchives/020612p48.shtml*
Infographic, p39
https://lpi.oregonstate.edu/mic/dietary-factors/phytochemicals/flavonoids
https://lpi.oregonstate.edu/mic/dietary-factors/phytochemicals/carotenoids
https://www.sciencedirect.com/topics/agricultural-and-biological-sciences/plant-pigments
http://www.whfoods.com/genpage.php?tname=nutrient&dbid=119
https://www.bhf.org.uk/informationsupport/heart-matters-magazine/nutrition/5-a-day/colourful-foods
https://www.wholekidsfoundation.org/assets/documents/better-bites-eat-a-rainbow.pdf

40–43 Opt for wholegrains
https://wholegrainscouncil.org/definition-whole-grain
https://paleofoundation.com/19-gluten-cross-reactive-foods/
Infographic, p41
https://wholegrainscouncil.org/sites/default/files/atoms/files/WGC-WhatIsWholeGrain.pdf

44–47 Find phytoestrogens
Infographic, p45
https://www.theveganrd.com/2014/01/soy-isoflavones-benefits-of-beans-and-mediterranean-foods-for-vegans/

56–57 An active lifestyle
Sternfeld B et al, "Efficacy of exercise for menopausal symptoms", *Menopause*. 2014, 21 (4): 330–8

https://pubmed.ncbi.nlm.nih.gov/23899828/

62–63 HRT and other medication
Menopause: diagnosis and treatment
https://www.nice.org.uk/guidance/ng23/chapter/Context
HRT and alternatives
https://www.guysandstthomas.nhs.uk/resources/patient-information/gynaecology/hormone-replacement-therapy.pdf
https://www.nhs.uk/conditions/hormone-replacement-therapy-hrt/
https://www.nhs.uk/conditions/hormone-replacement-therapy-hrt/alternatives/
Infographic, p63.
A Henderson, *Natural Menopause*, Dorling Kindersley, 2021, p211

64–65 Natural therapies and other practices
Johnson A et al, "Complementary and Alternative Medicine for Menopause", *Journal of Evidence Based Integrative Medicine*. 2019, 24:2515690X19829380
https://www.ncbi.nlm.nih.gov/pmc/articles/PMC6419242/
Acupuncture *https://www.evidencebasedacupuncture.org/acupuncture-menopause/*
https://acupuncture.org.uk/about-acupuncture/_fact-sheets/menopausal-symptoms/
Darsareh F et al, "Effect of aromatherapy massage on menopausal symptoms", *Menopause*, 2012, 19 (9): 995–9
https://pubmed.ncbi.nlm.nih.gov/22549173/
Complementary and alternative medicine for menopause
https://journals.sagepub.com/doi/pdf/10.1177/2515690X19829380
Natural remedies for hot flushes
http://www.menopause.org/for-women/menopauseflashes/menopause-symptoms-and-treatments/natural-remedies-for-hot-flashes
Fenugreek
Neal's Yard Remedies, *Complete Wellness*, Dorling Kindersley, 2018, p251

Acknowledgments

Author's dedication

To my grandmother and my son, whom I love so dearly. To all the wonderful midlife women who deserve a phenomenal second spring.

Author's acknowledgments

I am forever grateful to Dawn Henderson for entrusting me with this amazing project; to Claire Cross for making this book come to life, from ideas and concepts to a beautiful book; to Emma and Tom Forge, for their beautiful layouts and infographics; to Luke J. Albert and his team, for their stunning photographs. Also a big thank you to all the people who have worked on making this book available worldwide.

Publisher's acknowledgments

DK would like to thank: Severine Menem for her guidance and expertise. Also, Claire Wedderburn-Maxwell for proofreading, and Hilary Bird for indexing.
